HEALTH
HANDBOOK

HEALTH
HANDBOOK

by Louise Tenney, M.H.

Woodland Publishing
Pleasant Grove, UT

Health Handbook

Copyright © 1996 Louise Tenney

Woodland Publishing
P.O. Box 160
Pleasant Grove, Utah 84062

Contents

Notice to Reader

This herbal health book is not intended to prescribe or diagnose in any way. It is not meant to be a substitute for professional help. The intent is to offer historical uses of herbs. Those who are sick should consult their doctor.

Neither the author nor the publisher directly or indirectly dispense medical advice or prescribe the use of herbs as a form of treatment. The author and the publisher assume no responsibility if you prescribe for yourself without your doctor's approval.

Dedication

This book is dedicated to all those who have used *Today's Herbal Health.* In this way I can show my appreciation for the support you have given me. You have encouraged me to seek more and more knowledge about the use of herbs and their benefit to mankind.

Introduction

This handbook has been written as a guide to family health. Many people are turning to holistic healing which includes the physical, mental and spiritual aspects of the body. This book puts emphasis on the physical--using herbs, vitamins, minerals and supplements. Herbal food is emphasized because its healing properties are in tune with nature and therefore very beneficial to the human body.

There is an urgent need for enlightenment in this modern age on the uses of nature's herbal food. Herbalists see nature as a positive force in healing the body, and there herbs provide minerals, vitamins and nutrients that are in tune with the human body, therefore providing natural material for the body to heal itself.

Maintaining good health should be the goal of everyone. Herbs, vitamins, minerals and good food can become the daily weapon against illness. Herbs help to balance body chemistry to avoid disease. Herbs can provide energy and proper blood circulation to eliminate toxic accumulation and congestion that cause disease. Herbs help in digestion, assimilation and proper elimination. Herbs can be used in minor ailments and emergency aid as well as long-standing disease in acute or chronic conditions.

The last ten years have been a wonderful experience in meeting with thousands of people who have found health in the power of herbs.

AILMENTS

Acne

Acne can be caused from allergies, hormonal imbalance, stress, "the pill", and an excess intake of junk food causing an imbalanced body chemistry. The skin is the largest organ of elimination, and when the kidney and liver are backed up, excess waste is thrown off through the skin.

Herbal Combinations: Allergy, Blood Purifier, Bone Combination, Female or Prostate (to balance hormones), Liver, Lower Bowels.

Single Herbs: Alfalfa, *Aloe Vera,* Black Cohosh (balance hormones), *Black Walnut,* Burdock, Cascara Sagrada, Capsicum, *Chaparral,* Chickweed, *Dandelion, Dong Quai,* Echinacea, Ginseng, *Golden Seal,* Hops, *Kelp,* Lobelia, Oatstraw, Red Clover, Redmond Clay (external), Sarsaparilla, Scullcap, *White Oak Bark,* Yellow Dock.

Vitamins: A (up to 100,000 I.U. in beta carotene form every day for one month), B-complex (extra vitamin B2, B6, niacin, PABA, biotin), C (with bioflavonoids), and E.

Minerals: Calcium and magnesium (balanced), potassium, sulphur, selenium, zinc (as low as 20 mg. a day has helped to clear acne.

Amino Acids: Lysine, Tryptophan.

Supplements: Bee Pollen and Spirulina (RNA & DNA), Evening Primrose Oil, Black Currant Oil, Fish Lipids, Chlorophyll and Acidophilus; fresh juice fasting exercise with fresh air and sunshine; Peppermint Oil facial steam baths; use Redmond Clay facial scrub; Tea Tree Oil.

Abscess

This is an infection where pus collects in a part of the body. It can cause fever, tenderness and swelling. It is usually a local infection.

Herbal Combinations: Blood Purifier, Infection, Lower Bowel.

Single Herbs: *Black Walnut*, Burdock, Cayenne, Comfrey, Chaparral, Dandelion, *Echinacea*, Fenugreek, *Golden Seal*, Garlic, Kelp, *Pau D'Arco*, Rose Hips, Slippery Elm, Yellow Dock.

Vitamins: A (large amounts at first), B-complex (with pantothenic acid), vitamin C (with bioflavonoids), vitamins E (internally), vitamin E (externally--to heal after drained).

Minerals: Selenium, zinc.

Amino Acids: Free-form amino acids (speeds healing).

Supplements: Aloe Vera Juice (internally) and Aloe Vera Gel (externally), Acidophilus, Chlorophyll, Lecithin; extra pure water and liquids; poultice to draw out infections (three parts Golden Seal, two parts Black Walnut, two parts Slippery Elm, one part Comfrey, and add Aloe Vera Juice or pure water to make a paste); Black Ointment.

Aging

Premature aging is accelerated with bad diets and abuse of the body. It can cause chronic illness and lack of mental alertness. To help slow the aging process eat less food and exercise and more.

Herbal Combinations: Bone Combination, Chelation, Digestion, Endurance, Glands, Immune, Sex Rejuvenation.

Single Herbs: *Alfalfa,* Cayenne, *Damiana,* Dandelion, *Dong Quai,* Eyebright, False Unicorn, *Garlic,* Gentian, *Ginseng, Gotu Kola,* Hawthorn, Hops, Ho Shou-Wu, Kelp (Chelates metals), Lady's Slipper Licorice, Lobelia, Papaya, *Pau D'Arco, Red Clover,* Sarsaparilla, Yellow Dock, Yucca.

Vitamins: A, B-complex (extra choline), C (with bioflavonoids), E.

Minerals: Calcium and magnesium (balanced), iron (Dandelion and Yellow Dock), selenium, silicon, sulphur zinc.

Amino Acids: Arginine, Cysteine, Methionine (slows aging), Carnitine and Tyrosine (with vitamin B6 and C for assimilation to slow aging).

Supplements: Bee Pollen, Evening Primrose Oil, Black Currant Oil, Fish Oil Lipids, Lecithin (choline and inositol), Spirulina (RNA-DNA), Royal Jelly, Whey Powder or Raw Goat's Milk.

AIDS
(Acquired Immune Deficiency Syndrome)

AIDS affects the brain and nervous system. Everyone should be concerned about AIDS--it has been found in saliva and tears. It is a very serious and contagious disease. AIDS symptoms can lie dormant for up to ten years.

Herbal Combinations: Blood Purifier, Digestion, Infection, Immune, Liver, Lower Bowels.

Single Herbs: *Black Walnut,* Burdock, Cayenne, *Chaparral, Echinacea, Garlic,* Kelp, Marshmallow, *Pau D'Arco, Red Clover,* Sarsaparilla, Scullcap, Wormwood.

Vitamins: Multi-vitamins with extra vitamin A, B-complex, C (with bioflavonoids), D, and E.

Minerals: Multi-minerals with extra calcium, selenium, zinc.

Amino Acids: Free-form amino acids; Methionine, Cysteine and Taurine (work together as a team); Tryptophan (cleans blood).

Supplements: Acidophilus, Algin, Bee Pollen, Caprylic Acid, Evening Primrose Oil, Black Currant Oil, Lecithin, Spirulina, Wheat Grass Juice; 80% Raw Live Food; Green Drinks; Chlorophyll; Raw Food Diet.

Alcoholism

Alcoholism causes damage to the brain and liver. Therefore, nutrients are not assimilated. Alcohol leaches out vitamins and minerals. It can cause low blood sugar and/or a deficiency in calcium, B-complex and magnesium.

Herbal Combinations: Digestion, Glands, Heart, Liver, Nerves.

Single Herbs: *Alfalfa,* Black Cohosh, Black Walnut, *Chaparral,* Dandelion, Echinacea, Garlic, Ginseng, *Golden Seal,* Gota Kola, Hawthorn, *Hops,* Kelp, Licorice, Lobelia, Passion Flower, *Red Clover, Scullcap, Valerian,* Wood Betony, Wormwood, Yellow Dock.

Vitamins: Multi-vitamins, extra A (up to 100,000 i.u. in beta carotene form every day for one month), B-complex, vitamin C (with bioflavonoids), pantothenic acid (to help in adrenal exhaustion), choline and inositol to break up fat in the liver.

Minerals: Multi-minerals, extra calcium and magnesium (balanced), selenium, zinc.

Amino Acids: Glutamine (helps stop cravings), Methionine (protects kidneys and liver), Cysteine, Tyrosine.

Supplements: Evening Primrose Oil, Rice Bran Syrup (easy assimilation), Acidophilus, Chlorophyll, Herbal Teas.

Allergies

Incomplete digestion can throw toxins back into the bloodstream and cause allergic reactions. Stress, worry and fear can cause allergies by weakening the immune system. A common allergy is hay fever (swollen, itchy eyes and runny nose).

Herbal Combinations: Allergy, Bone Combinations, Digestion, Lungs, Lower Bowel.

Single Herbs: Alfalfa, *Burdock*, Chaparral, Chickweed, *Comfrey,* Dandelion, *Echinacea*, Eyebright, Fenugreek, Gentian, *Golden Seal,* Gotu Kola, Hops Ho-Shou-Wu, Irish Moss, Lobelia, *Ma Huang* (natural antihistamine), Myrrh, Parsley, Red Raspberry, Scullcap, Wood Betony, Wormwood, Yellow dock.

Vitamins: Multi-vitamins with extra A, B-complex (pantothenic acid, B6, B12), C.

Minerals: Multi-minerals with extra calcium and magnesium (balanced), manganese, potassium, zinc.

Amino Acids: Histidine, Isoleucine, Tryptophan, Tyrosine.

Supplements: Bee Pollen, Acidophilus (milk free); Bentonite, Black Currant Oil, Chinese Essential Oils, Fish Oil Lipids, Primrose Oil, Rice Bran Syrup, Royal-Jelly, Glucomannan.

Supplements: Bee Pollen, Acidophilus (milk free); Bentonite, Black Currant Oil, Chinese Essential Oils, Fish Oil Lipids, Primrose Oil, Rice Bran Syrup, Royal-

Jelly, Glucomannan.

Anemia

Anemia can cause fatigue, paleness, loss of appetite, headaches, frequent infections, general weakness and irrational behavior. Poor assimilation of vitamin B12 and iron can contribute to anemia, therefore hydrochloric acid and calcium are needed to assimilate vitamin B12 and iron. Dandelion and Yellow Dock will help build rich red blood.

Herbal Combinations: Anemia, Blood Purifier, Digestion, Liver.

Single Herbs: *Alfalfa*, Barberry, Black Walnut, Burdock, Cayenne, Chaparral, *Dandelion*, Dong Quai, Echinacea, Garlic, *Gentian*, Ginger, Golden Seal, Hawthorn, *Kelp*, Lobelia, Red Clover, Sarsaparilla, Watercress, *Yellow Dock.*

Vitamins: A, B-complex (extra B6, B12, folic acid), PABA and pantothenic acid), C (with bioflavonoids—aids in digestion of iron), E (carries oxygen to the cells).

Minerals: Calcium and magnesium (balanced), copper, iron, zinc.
Amino Acids: Histidine, Lysine, lsoleucine.

Supplements: Beet Powder, Chlorophyll, Evening Primrose Oil, Blackstrap Molasses, Apricots, Spirulina, Sesame Seeds (contains vitamin T—which helps in blood coagulation and the forming of platelets); good for anemia and hemophilia.

Anorexia Nervosa

Anorexia is self-induced starvation and is characterized by broken blood vessels in the face, underweight, weakness and dizziness. Bulimia is a constant excessive insatiable appetite followed by self-induced vomiting. Both bulimia and anorexia may be symptoms of a disease and/or psychotic problems.

Herbal Combinations: Allergies, Digestion, Glands, Hypoglycemia, Nerves.

Single Herbs: Black Cohosh, Black Walnut, Burdock, Catnip, *Chamomile*, Chaparral, *Dandelion,* Echinacea, Ginger, Ginseng, Gotu Kola, Hops, Ho Shou Wu, *Kelp, Lady's Slipper, Licorice,* Lobelia, Papaya, Passion Flower, Peppermint, *Scullcap, Red Clover, Wild Yam,* Wood Betony, *Yellow Dock.*

Vitamins: A, B-complex, C (with bioflavonoids), D, E.

Minerals: Multi-minerals with calcium and magnesium (balanced), potassium (lost during vomiting and excess laxatives), sodium, zinc (excreted quickly in starvation).
Amino Acids: Free-form amino acids; all amino acids are needed to build healthy cells.

Supplements: Evening Primrose Oil (vitamin F), Black Currant Oil, Fish Oil Lipids, Acidophilus, Green Drinks (chlorophyll).

Appetite

Appetite can be lost due to sickness. Normal appetite should return as health increases.

Herbal Combinations: Digestion, Glands, Nerves.

Single Herbs: Alfalfa, *Aloe Vera*, Catnip, *Chamomile*, Dandelion, Gentian, Ginger, Golden Seal, Hops, *Papaya*, Parsley, Passion Flower, *Peppermint*, Red Clover, Safflowers, Saffron, Scullcap, Slippery Elm, Thyme, Watercress, Yarrow.

Vitamins: A, B-complex, C (with bioflavonoids), D, E.

Minerals: Calcium and magnesium zinc.

Amino Acids: Free-form amino acids.

Supplements: Spirulina.

Arteriosclerosis

Arteriosclerosis is a disease that can cause strokes, high blood pressure, angina and heart problems. It is a result of fatty deposits that collect on the inner walls of the arteries.

Herbal Combinations: Blood Purifier, Bone Combinations, Heart, Chelation, Lower Bowels.

Single Herbs: *Alfalfa*, Aloe Vera, Black Walnut, Burdock, Capsicum, Chaparral, Comfrey, Echinacea, Garlic, Golden Seal, Hawthorn, Horsetail, Juniper Berries, Irish Moss, *Kelp*, Licorice, Marshmallow, *Pau D'Arco*, Red Clover, Slippery Elm, Watercress, Yellow Dock.

Vitamins: Multi-vitamin, B-complex (extra B6 and niacin), C (with bioflavonoids), E, choline, inositol (found in lecithin).

Minerals: Calcium, magnesium, chromium, selenium, zinc.

Amino Acids: Alanine (reduces cholesterol when combines with Arginine and Glycine), Carnitine, Cysteine, Glutamine, Methionine (prevents accumulation of fat in liver), Taurine.

Supplements: Lecithin, Evening Primrose Oil, Black Currant Oil, Co-Enzyme Q10, EPA-Fish Oil Lipids.

Arthritis

Arthritis is inflammation of the joints. Inflammation of the joints can also be found in bursitis, gout, tennis elbow, hips and shoulders. Arthritis is caused by deposits of crystallized uric acid in the joints—causing redness and pain. Checking for allergies can be helpful. A diet of no red meat, white flour, white sugar, salt, citrus fruit, and nightshade family (tomatoes, potatoes, green peppers, eggplant) is helpful for relief of arthritis.

Herbal Combinations: Arthritis, Blood Purifier, Bone Combination, Comfrey and Pepsin, Digestion, Nerve, Pain.

Single Herbs: *Alfalfa,* Aloe Vera, Brigham Tea, Burdock, Capsicum, Chaparral, Comfrey, Dandelion, *Devil's Claw,* Dulse, Garlic, Hydrangea, Kelp, Parsley, Papaya, Saffron, Red Clover, Watercress, *White Willow, Yucca.*

Vitamins: A, B-complex (extra B6, B12, niacin, pantothenic), C (with bioflavonoids), E.

Minerals: Calcium and magnesium (balance), selenium, silicon manganese and zinc.

Amino Acids: Free form amino acids, Cystine (works with pantothenic acid in arthritis treatment), Histidine (removes heavy metals), Phenylalanine (for pain).

Supplements: Distilled Water, Green Drinks, Juices (carrot and celery), Co-Enzyme Ql0, Fish Oil Lipids, Evening Primrose Oil, Black Currant Oil, Chinese Essential Oils, Rice Bran Syrup, Tea Tree Oil.

Asthma

For treatment of asthma, avoid sulfites (found in salads, frozen shrimp, potatoes, baked goods, sausage and wines). It also helps to eliminate mucus forming foods such as dairy products, white sugar and white flour products.

Herbal Combinations: Allergies, Digestion, Lungs, Nerves, Lower Bowels.

Single Herbs: Alfalfa, Aloe Vera, Bayberry, Black Cohosh, Brigham Tea, Burdock, *Capsicum,* Chaparral, *Cascara Sagrada,* Chickweed, *Comfrey,* Dandelion, Echinacea, Eyebright, *Fenugreek, Garlic,* Ginseng, Golden Seal, Gotu Kola, *Hops,* Horsetail, Ho Shou-Wu, Licorice, *Lobelia,* Marshmallow, Ma Huang, Mullein, Oat Straw, Pau D'Arco, Red Clover, Rose Hips, Scullcap, *Slippery Elm,* Valerian, White Willow, Wood Betony, Yarrow, Yellow Dock.

Vitamins: A, B-complex (extra B6, B12, PABA,

pantothenic acid), C (with bioflavonoids), E (low doses to start).

Minerals: Calcium and magnesium (balance), manganese, potassium, zinc, herbal potassium.

Amino Acids: Free form amino acids (builds new tissues), Glutathione, Histidine, Isoleucine (regulates glands).

Supplements: Chlorophyll, Lemon Juice, Pure Water, Juice Fast, RNA-DNA Foods, Sardines, Spirulina, Bee Pollen; Tincture of Lobelia for emergency; Colon Cleanse have helped many people; Black Currant Oil or Evening Primrose Oil, Fish Oil Lipids, Tea Tree Oil.

Backache

Backache could be a result of constipation, back strain, kidney infection, stress or calcium deficiency.

Herbal Combinations: Bone Combination, Digestion, Lower Bowels, Nerves, Pain.

Single Herbs: Alfalfa, Aloe Vera, Burdock, *Comfrey,* Dandelion, Hops, *Horsetail,* Lady's Slipper, *Oatstraw,* Scullcap, *Slippery Elm,* White Willow.

Vitamins: A, B-complex, C, D, E.

Minerals: Calcium and magnesium (balance), manganese, silicon, zinc.

Amino Acids: Phenylalanine (for pain).

Supplements: Cleansing Fasts, Herbal Creams (for external use), Pau D'Arco Lotion, Chinese Essential Oils; Peppermint Oil, Tea Tree Oil.

Bad Breath

Bad breath could be a result of gum or tooth decay, constipation, colon congestion, poor diet, excess smoking or liver problems.

Herbal Combinations: Blood Purifier, Digestion, Liver, Lower Bowels.

Single Herbs: *Alfalfa*, Aloe Vera, Capsicum, *Cascara Sagrada*, Cloves, Echinacea, Irish Moss, *Kelp*, Golden Seal, Myrrh, *Parsley*, Peppermint, Watercress.

Vitamins: A, B-complex (daily), C (with bioflavonoids—daily), E.

Minerals: Multi-minerals, extra potassium, selenium, zinc.

Supplements: Liquid Chlorophyll, Acidophilus, Green Drinks; Short Raw Food Diet; Fresh Lemon Juice in Pure Water; Dental Floss.

Baldness

Baldness can be inherited. It can also be caused by a lack of minerals, drugs, poor diet, stress, or poor circulation. It can be helpful to eliminate white sugar and white flour products for treatment of baldness. Many individuals who have cleaned their blood and changed to a vegetarian diet have grown thick hair.

Herbal Combinations: Blood Purification, Hair, Skin and Nails, Heart (for circulation), General Cleanser, Glands, Lower Bowels.

Single Herbs: *Aloe Vera,* Bayberry, Black Walnut, Burdock, Capsicum, Comfrey, Chamomile, Echinacea, Garlic, Ginger, Ginseng, Hawthorn, *Horsetail, Jojoba, Kelp, Oatstraw,* Sage, Sarsaparilla, White Oak.

Vitamins: A, B-complex, C, D, E, extra PABA, biotin and inositol.

Minerals: Calcium and magnesium (balance), manganese, iron, silicon, sulphur, zinc.

Amino Acids: L-Cysteine (improves color and texture), L-Methionine (prevents hair loss—take with vitamin B6 and C for proper absorption).

Supplements: Lecithin, Evening Primrose Oil or Black Currant Oil, Linseed Oil; use Slant Board; hair shampoo containing Caprylic Acid; raw seeds and nuts, raw juices; use sprouts; stimulate hair with pure Olive Oil; drink Pau D'Arco and Red Clover Tea.

Bedwetting

Bedwetting may be caused by emotional upsets, infections, or extreme tiredness. In order to help stop bedwetting, stay away from chocolate, sugar products, milk, wheat and white flour products.

Herbal Combinations: Bladder and Kidneys, Bone Combination, Glands, Nerves.

Single Herbs: Buchu, Cornsilk, Dandelion, *Hops,* Marshmallow, *Oatstraw, Parsley,* Scullcap, St. Johnswort, *Uva Ursi.*

Vitamins: A, B-complex (nerves), C (during day—kills toxins), E.

Minerals: Calcium (calms nerves) and magnesium (balance), potassium, zinc.

Amino Acids: Free-form amino acids (deficiency has been linked with bedwetting).

Supplements: Bee Pollen, Evening Primrose Oil, Black Currant Oil, Chlorophyll.

Bladder

Bladder ailments may include infections, cystitis or kidney infections, blood in urine, and painful or frequent urination. For treatment of bladder ailments, avoid coffee, cola drinks and alcohol—drink pure water and try juice fasts. It can be helpful to eliminate chocolate and mucus forming foods.

Herbal Combinations: Bladder and Kidneys, Digestion, Infections, Glands.

Single Herbs: Alfalfa, Burdock, *Cornsilk,* Dandelion, Garlic, Golden Seal, *Juniper Berries,* Kelp, Marshmallow, *Parsley,* Pau D'Arco, Red Raspberry, Rose Hips, *Uva Ursi,* Yarrow.

Vitamins: A, B-complex (extra B6, pantothenic acid, choline), C (with bioflavonoids), E.

Minerals: Calcium and magnesium (balance), manganese, potassium, selenium, zinc.

Amino Acids: L-Cysteine, L-Methionine.

Supplements: Liquid Chlorophyll, Acidophilus, Flaxseed Tea, Green Drinks.

Bleeding-Hemorrhage

Bleeding generally refers to external loss of blood. Hemorrhage usually refers to internal rupture of a blood vessel. Common bleeding ailments are bleeding gums or nose bleeds (rutin deficiency). Serious bleeding can usually be stopped by applying direct pressure—after which professional assistance should be obtained.

Herbal Combinations: Anemia, Bone Combination, Hair-Skin-Nails, Heart and Blood Pressure, Infection.

Single Herbs: Alfalfa (contains Vitamin K), Bayberry, Blackberry, Bugleweed, *Capsicum* (for both internal and external bleeding—1 teaspoon in a glass of warm water), Comfrey, *Dong Qua*i (internal), Ephedra (internal), *False Unicorn* (uterine), Golden Seal (nose and uterine—internal and external), *Horsetail* (internal), Juniper, Marshmallow (bladder), *Mullein* (bowel and lungs), Pau D'Arco (all kinds), *White Oak Bark* (nose, urinary and uterine— internal),Yarrow.

Vitamins: A, B-complex, C (with bioflavonoids), K

(alfalfa and chlorophyll).

Minerals: Calcium and magnesium (balance), trace minerals (such as selenium and zinc).

Amino Acids: Isoleucine (necessary for hemoglobin formation), Leucine (essential for blood development).

Supplements: Aloe Vera (prevents scarring), Vitamin E (prevents scarring—both internally and externally), Liquid Chlorophyll.

Blood, Impure

The liver and bowels are usually in need of cleansing when the blood is impure. Many diseases (such as gangrene) stem from toxic blood as well as infections. Juice cleansing is a good treatment for impure blood.

Herbal Combinations: Blood Purifier, Bone Combination, Immune, Liver and Gallbladder, General Cleanser, Lower Bowels.

Single Herbs: Alfalfa, Bayberry, Black Walnut, *Burdock* (good blood cleanser), Butchers Broom, *Cascara Sagrada, Chaparral,* Dandelion, Echinacea, Fenugreek, Garlic, Golden Seal, Kelp, Licorice, Pau D'Arco, *Red Clover,* Sarsaparilla, Yellow Dock, Yarrow.

Vitamins: A, C and E.

Minerals: Selenium, zinc.

Amino Acids: Isoleucine (essential for healthy blood),

Arginine (purifies blood).

Supplements: Barley Juice, Chlorophyll, Liquid, Wheat Grass; Raw vegetables are needed; Echinacea Extract.

Boils

A cleansing diet, along with exercise and fresh air speeds the healing of boils. Enemas are often indicated in the treatment of boils. Honey with small amounts of comfrey powder applied to the boil will help bring it to a head. Slippery Elm powder mixed with aloe vera juice is also very healing.

Herbal Combinations: Blood Purifier, Bone Combinations, Digestion, General Cleanser, Lower Bowels.

Single Herbs: Aloe Vera, Black Walnut, *Burdock,* Capsicum, *Chaparral,* Comfrey, Dandelion, *Echinacea,* Kelp, Lobelia, Mullein, *Pau D'Arco, Red Clover,* Yellow Dock.

Vitamins: A, C (with bioflavonoids), E (up to 800 I.U. a day).

Minerals: Multi-minerals, extra calcium and magnesium (balance), silicon, selenium, zinc (50 to 100 mg. per day).

Amino Acids: Free-form amino acids.

Supplements: Liquid Chlorophyll; Flaxseed Poultice

and Clay Packs; Chinese Oil Formula; drink Red Clover and Pau D'Arco Tea (to clean blood); Black Ointment, Echinacea Extract, Tea Tree Oil.

Brain

Brain function depends on a healthy liver. Good digestion is needed for proper brain function. Reading and learning worthwhile things stretches the brain. It is also helpful to use a slant board--extra blood to head.

Herbal Combinations: Heart, Glands, Digestion, Liver, Lower Bowels, Nerves.

Single Herbs: Alfalfa, Black Cohosh, *Burdock,* Capsicum, Chaparral, Echinacea, Garlic, Ginger, *Ginseng,* Golden Seal, *Gotu Kola,* Hops, Ho Shou-Wu, Lobelia, *Licorice,* Mistletoe, Rosemary, Red Clover, Scullcap, Watercress, *Wood Betony,* Yellow Dock.

Vitamins: A, B-complex (with extra thiamine, B6, niacin, B15).

Minerals: Multi-minerals, extra selenium, zinc.

Amino Acids: L-Arginine, L-Tyrosine (for anxiety and depression), L-Glutamine (improves emotional stress and mental function), Tryptophan (for relaxation), Phenylalanine and Valine (for mental vigor), and Leucine (stimulates brain function).

Supplements: Lecithin, RNA-nutrients, sardines, spirulina, chlorella and bee pollen; raw goat's milk builds brain and the nervous system.

Bronchitis

Bronchitis is a very common disease. It can be caused by polluted air or smoking--which weakens the lungs. Coughing, wheezing and spitting up mucus along with difficult breathing are common symptoms. Allergies are often connected with bronchitis. The body's resistance is depleted rapidly when it has bronchitis. Hot drinks are suggested to encourage perspiration. Lobelia extract taken every hour has helped to loosen congestion. A change of diet to more alkaline foods (avoid milk products--except raw goat's milk) can be helpful. Cleansing fasts can help heal bronchitis more rapidly.

Herbal Combinations: Allergy, Blood Cleanser, Digestion, Lower Bowels, Lungs, Nerves.

Single Herbs: *Boneset (helps aches),* Capsicum, *Cascara Sagrada, Comfrey,* Echinacea and Golden Seal Extract, Eucalyptus, Garlic (Antiseptic), Ginger, Licorice, *Lobelia (chest constrictor),* Ma Huang, *Marshmallow,* Mullein, *Pau D'Arco, Slippery Elm.*

Vitamins: A (up to 100,000 I.U. in beta carotene form for one month), B-complex (speeds healing), C (with bioflavonoids), D, E.

Minerals: Multi-minerals, extra iron (Dandelion and Yellow Dock), manganese, silicon, sodium, zinc (lozenges).

Amino Acids: Free-form amino acids (use between meals), extra Cysteine, Arginine and Ornithine.

Supplements: Hot Lemon Juice with Pure Maple Syrup; Hot Herbal Drink made with Roasted Barley, Malt, Chicory and Rye; Liquid Chlorophyll, Royal Jelly with Dong Quai, or Bee Propolis; Zinc Gluconate Lozenges.

Bruises

Increased bruising may be a result of anemia, malnutrition, overweight, and/or lack of vitamins and minerals. Too much aspirin can also cause increased bruising.

Herbal Combinations: Blood Cleanser, Bone Combination, Digestion.

Single Herbs: Alfalfa (contains vitamin K), *Black Walnut,* Capsicum, *Comfrey,* Dandelion, Dong Quai, Ginger, Hawthorn, Hops, *Horsetail, Kelp,* Lady's Slipper, Lobelia, Marshmallow, *Rose Hips,* Scullcap, *Slippery Elm,* St. Johnswort, *White Oak,* Yellow Dock.

Vitamins: Calcium and magnesium (balance), iron (Yellow dock and Dandelion or liquid chlorophyll), zinc.

Amino Acids: Free-form amino acids (between meals), Cystine.

Supplements: Liquid Chlorophyll; Poultice of Comfrey and Black Walnut mixed with Aloe Vera Juice (externally); Sesame Seeds (contains vitamin T, which helps build healthy blood platelets); Black Currant Oil and Redmond Clay.

Bruxism

Bruxism is teeth grinding. It is related to low adrenal function, and is often seen in those with hypoglycemia. Mercury leaking from the teeth can be a cause of bruxism. It happens during sleep--a person is not aware of bruxism taking place. It is possible to lose teeth if it's not caught in time. It is helpful to avoid sweet sugar products--especially just before retiring to bed.

Herbal Combinations: Bone Combinations, Glands, Heart, Nerves.

Single Herbs: Alfalfa, Black Walnut (mineral balancer), Burdock, Capsicum, Chaparral, *Comfrey,* Echinacea, Garlic, *Gotu Kola, Hops,* Horsetail, Ho Shou-Wu, Kelp, *Lady's Slipper,* Licorice, Lobelia, Marshmallow, Mistletoe, Oatstraw, *Passion Flower, Scullcap,* Slippery Elm, Red Clover, Watercress, *Wood Betony,* Yellow Dock.

Vitamins: Multi-vitamins, extra B-complex (extra B6, pantothenic acid), C (with bioflavonoids), E.

Minerals: Multi-minerals, extra calcium and magnesium (balance), sodium and potassium (balance), selenium, silicon, zinc.

Amino Acids: Tryptophan (with vitamin B6, C, calcium).

Supplements: Chlorophyll, Bee Pollen, Rice Bran Syrup.

Bulimia

Bulimia is abnormal increase in appetite and anorexia is self-induced starvation. It is very dangerous because it can destroy peristaltic action, ruin teeth from strong gastric juices caused by vomiting, cause osteoporosis and weaken the heart. Bulimics generally eat normal meals, but then binge on foods that are high to be "forbidden"-- high fat and sugar foods. Purging is followed with diuretics, laxatives or forced vomiting. Laxatives are often used excessively--up to fifty or sixty a day--and can be very dangerous. Bulimics suffer from fatigue, headaches, heart palpitations, pain, dysfunctions and muscle weakness.

Herbal Combinations: Bone Combinations, Digestion, Energy and Fitness, Glands, Heart and Blood Pressure, Immune, Nerve and Relaxant, Potassium, Stress.

Single Herbs: *Alfalfa*, Black Cohosh, Black Walnut, Catnip, *Chamomile*, Ginger, Ginseng (men), Gotu Kola, *Hops*, Ho Shou-Wu, Kelp, *Lady's Slipper*, Licorice, *Lobelia*, Papaya, Passion Flower, Peppermint, Scullcap, Red Clover, Wild Yam *Wood Betony*, Yellow Dock.

Vitamins: Multi-vitamins, extra B-complex (extra B6, B12), C (with bioflavonoids), E.

Minerals: Multi-minerals with extra calcium and magnesium (balance), manganese, potassium, selenium, silicon, sodium, zinc (zinc deficiency has been linked with bulimia and anorexia nervosa).

Amino Acids: Free-form amino acids.

Supplements: Acidophilus, Liquid Chlorophyll, Rice Bran Syrup.

Burns

There are three basic types of burns--first degree burns which cause redness, second degree burns which cause redness and blister, and third degree burns which cause destruction of the skin and underlying muscles. It is helpful to increase intake of fluids in treatment of burns. Ice water applied to infected are can draw out heat and ease pain. Vitamin E applied immediately to burns can alleviate pain and prevent blistering.

Herbal Combinations: Bone (increases healing), Infections, Nerve and Relaxant.

Single Herbs: *Aloe Vera,* Chickweed, Comfrey, Garlic, *Horsetail*, Marshmallow (acid or fire burns), Oatstraw, Red Clover, *Slippery Elm,* Witch Hazel, Yarrow.

Vitamins: A (100,000 I.U. daily for a month), C (with bioflavonoids), B-complex (extra B12), E (used internally and externally).

Minerals: Multi-minerals (burns heal faster with minerals), calcium and magnesium (balance), potassium, sodium, selenium, zinc.

Amino Acids: Free-form amino acids (between meals), Cysteine.

Supplements: Aloe Vera on first degree burns(after healing can be used on 2nd and 3rd degree burns to prevent scarring); Evening Primrose Oil or Black Currant

Oil, Chinese essential oils, Redmond Clay, Tea Tree Oil.

Cancer

Cancer is a serious, fast-growing disease. Cancer is linked to poor diet, stress and environmental pollution. Cancer is affected by change of diet and emotional health. The immune system needs to be strengthened and there needs to be a balance in all areas of life in order to prevent cancer. Eat foods rich in B17, and use pure water, grains, nuts, seeds, brown rice, millet, fruits and raw vegetables to help strengthen the immune system.

Herbal Combinations: Blood Purifier, Bone Combination, Candida, Cleansing, Digestion, General Cleanser, Glands, Immune, Lower Bowels, Nerves and Relaxant, Potassium, (Comfrey and Pepsin dissolve dead meat cells).

Single Herbs: *Burdock, Chaparral,* Dandelion, Echinacea, *Garlic,* Golden Seal, Kelp, Parsley, Pau D'Arco, *Red Clover (Red Clover Blend Tea),* Yellow Dock.

Vitamins: Multi-vitamins needed daily with extra vitamin A, C (with bioflavonoids), B-complex (with extra niacin, choline, B12, B17), E.

Minerals: Multi-minerals with extra calcium and magnesium (balance), potassium, selenium, zinc.

Amino Acids: Free-form amino acids (between meals), extra Cysteine, Methionine (contains sulphur and selenium), Lysine (may lessen incidence of cancer), Tyrosine.

Supplements: Macrobiotic diet has been successful for some people; No meat and high fiber diet is also successful; Lecithin, Acidophilus, Liquid Chlorophyll, Evening Primrose Oil or Black Currant Oil; Garlic daily; Carrot Juice, Cabbage Juice, Raw Beet, Wheat Grass Juice; Black Ointment (for skin cancer), Garlic Oil and Fish Oil Lipids.

Candida Albicans

Candidiasis is a modern day plague, stemming from the antibiotic age. It is a fungus outgrowth. The elimination of antibiotics, birth control pills and all drugs is necessary for treatment of candida. It is also necessary to change the diet--stop eating the foods that feed the yeast. It is helpful to build the immune system by using herbs, vitamins, minerals, amino acids and other necessary supplements. (See booklet *Candida Albicans, A Nutritional Approach*, by Louise Tenney).

Herbal Combinations: Blood Purifier, Candida Combination, Cleansing Combination, General Cleanser, Immune, Nerve and Relaxant, Stress.

Single Herbs: Alfalfa, *Black Walnut,* Burdock, Capsicum, *Chaparral,* Dandelion, Dong Quai, *Echinacea, Garlic,* Hops, Horsetail, Kelp, Lady's Slipper, Licorice, Mistletoe, Passion Flower, *Pau D'Arco, Red Clover,* Sarsaparilla, Scullcap, Valerian, White Oak, Yellow Dock.

Vitamins: A, B-complex (yeast free), C (with bioflavonoids), E.

Amino Acids: Free-form amino acids (between meals).

Supplements: Acidophilus, Evening Primrose Oil, Black Currant Oil, Caprylic Acid, Psyllium Hulls, Tea Tree Oil.

Canker Sores

Allergies, stress, and unbalanced body chemistry can cause mouth disorders such as cold sores, sore gums, pyorrhea and thrush. Rinsing the mouth with Golden Seal, Black Walnut and White Oak Bark will help heal the canker sores, firm the gums and stop infections.

Herbal Combinations: Blood Purifier, Ulcers.

Single Herbs: Aloe Vera, Burdock, *Capsicum, Comfrey,* Chaparral, Echinacea, *Garlic, Golden Seal,* Gotu Kola, Hawthorn, Lady's Slipper, Lobelia, Myrrh, Oatstraw, Red Raspberry, Scullcap, *White Oak Bark,* Wood Betony, Yellow Dock.

Vitamins: A, B-complex (extra B12, pantothenic acid), C (with bioflavonoids), E.

Minerals: Calcium and magnesium (balance), iron, phosphorus, selenium, zinc.

Amino Acids: L-Lysine.

Supplements: Make a paste with Golden Seal, Black Walnut and Aloe Vera Juice and put on infected area; Acidophilus, Liquid Chlorophyll, Tea Tree Oil, Chinese

Essential Oils (externally); at first sign, use ice for thirty minutes and alternate Vitamin A and cheweable Vitamin C on canker sore.

Childhood Diseases

Childhood diseases include chicken pox, measles, mumps, rheumatic fever and scarlet fever. During chicken pox avoid aspirin--could cause Reye's Syndrome. Measles causes a skin rash. Mumps is a contagious viral infection and can spread to ovaries, pancreas, testicles and the nervous system. Rheumatic fever is a strep infection and can affect the brain, heart and joints. Scarlet fever is a strep infection with sore throat, swollen lymph glands and cough. Scarlatina is a mild form of scarlet fever.

Herbal Combinations: Blood Purifier, Bone Combinations, Cleansing, Colds and Flu, Immune, Insomnia, Pain.

Single Herbs: Alfalfa (hot tea), *Catnip (tea and for enema) Chamomile,* Capsicum, *Cascara Sagrada (open bowels),* Eyebright, Echinacea, *Garlic, Ginger (baths),* Golden Seal (relieves itching), Hops (relaxes nerves), *Lady's Slipper, Lobelia,* Mullein, Pau D'Arco, Peppermint (tea), Pleurisy Root, Red Clover, Red Raspberry, Rose Hips, Safflower, *Scullcap,* Yarrow, Yellow Dock.

Vitamins: A, B-complex (depleted fast in illness—rice bran syrup is best), C (with bioflavonoids).

Minerals: Multi-minerals (liquid) extra calcium and magnesium (balance), potassium, selenium, zinc.

Amino Acids: Free-form amino acids (liquid--to repair tissues), Methionine (especially for rheumatic fever).

Supplements: Liquids in the form of Chlorophyll, Herbal Drinks, Lemon-Lime Aloe Vera Drink, Raspberry Tea Combination; Liquid or Powdered Vitamin C; Use Raw Applesauce for use with herbs; Use Garlic with Vitamin C; for fever (nature's way to destroy toxins), use of White Willow, Catnip Tea, Hops and Scullcap will help reduce fevers; keep bowels open with enemas or herbal laxatives; drink liquids frequently to prevent dehydration; Lobelia Extract helps with fevers; Black Currant Oil or Evening Primrose Oil, Echinacea Extract, Instant Vitamins.

Chemical Poisoning

There are chemical additives everywhere--air, food and water. It is concentrated in meat, seeping into the water from crop spraying, nuclear fallout, and sewage. It is best to eat wholesome foods which act as a protection against build-up of chemicals. Suggested foods are whole grains, beans, fruits and vegetables.

Herbal Combinations: Blood Purifier, Bone Combination, Candida, Chelation, Digestion, General Cleanser, Glands, Immune, Lower Bowels, Potassium, Stress, Thyroid.

Single Herbs: Alfalfa, Aloe Vera, *Bugleweed, Chaparral,* Comfrey and Fenugreek (lungs), *Echinacea* *(glands)*, *Garlic*, Horseradish, Horsetail Kelp (natural iodine), *Pau D'Arco, Red Clover, Yellow Dock.*

Vitamins: A, B-complex, C (with bioflavonoids), E.

Minerals: Multi-minerals, extra selenium, zinc.

Amino Acids:' Sulphur amino acids, L-Cysteine Glutathione, Histidine, L-Methionine.

Supplements: Algin, Chlorophyll, Hydrated Bentonote (must use with enemas), Pectin, Wheat Grass: Hydrochloric Acid is necessary in the blood to fight chemicals, infections and maintain the acid-alkaline balance; Algin, Fish Oil Lipids, Echinacea Extract. Redmond Clay; Nutritional Fiber Supplement.

Celiac Disease

Celiac disease are most often inherited. It is an intestinal problem caused by gluten intolerance. The lining of the small intestine is damaged and foods are not digested or absorbed and this causes malabsorption of nutrients. Foods that give the most problems are barley, oats, rye and wheat. Celiac disease causes diarrhea, stomach pain, gas, anemia and malnutrition.

Herbal Combinations: Blood Purifier, Anemia, Digestion (enzymes).

Single Herbs: Alfalfa, Dandelion, Kelp, Papaya, *Saffron (for digestion)*, Slippery Elm, Yellow Dock.

Vitamins: Multi-vitamins (liquid), B-complex (extra

folic acid, B12--rice bran syrup), C (with bioflavonoids--liquid), iron.

Minerals: Calcium and magnesium (balance).

Amino Acids: Free-form amino acids (liquid).

Supplements: Chlorophyll (liquid), Glucomannan (colon cleanse--not absorbed by intestines but provides bulk); use millet, buckwheat, brown rice.

Colds and Flu

Frequent colds, flu, and pneumonia could be allergies to milk, wheat products or food additives, etc. Keep the body clean--germs spread through handshakes. Don't suppress colds--it's the body's way of getting rid of the toxins and infections. Coughs and hoarseness with mucus (Comfrey and Fenugreek, Licorice), Dry cough (open capsule of Slippery Elm and mix with juice and let it coat the throat), Croup (Tincture of Lobelia under tongue and rub on spine), Warm Catnip or Chamomile Tea.

Herbal Combinations: Allergy, comfrey and Fenugreek (breaks up mucus), Colds and Flu, Infection, Lower Bowel, Nerves and Relaxant, Potassium.

Single Herbs: *Alfalfa Tea,* Aloe Vera, Capsicum, Comfrey, Dandelion, *Fenugreek, Garlic, Ginger (settles stomach), Golden Seal, Kelp,* Licorice, *Lobelia, Marshmallow,* Ma Huang, Mullein, Passion Flower, Red Raspberry, *Rose Hips, Slippery Elm (for coughs and also heals throat).*

Vitamins: A (in beta carotene form--high amounts at first), C (with bioflavonoids), B-complex (depleted fast in illness).

Minerals: Calcium and magnesium (balance--builds bloods and sustains nerves), potassium, selenium, zinc.

Amino Acids: Free-form amino acids, Lysine (helps in viral infections), L-Carnitine, L-Cysteine.

Supplements: Green Drinks, Vegetable Broths, liquids in Herbal Drinks, Hot Herbal Teas (Alfalfa, Peppermint), Lemon-Lime Aloe Vera Drink, Raspberry Tea Combination, liquid or powder Vitamin C in drinks; use raw applesauce with herbs for children; Rice Bran Syrup; cold extremities can be balanced with Capsicum and Lobelia (restores balance between the autonomic nervous system--returning heat to the body); Black Currant Oil, Chinese Essential Oils, Garlic Oil, Echinacea Extract, Licorice Lozenges are effective, Peppermint Oil, Tea Tree Oil.

Colitis

Common causes of colitis are stress, allergies, faulty diet and/or poor digestion. Colitis is inflammation of the colon which causes diarrhea alternating with constipation.

Herbal Combinations: Bone Combination, Comfrey and Pepsin, Colitis, Digestion, Lower Bowels, Ulcers.

Single Herbs: *Aloe Vera (healing),* Alfalfa (vitamin K is needed), Dandelion, Garlic, *Hops,* Kelp, Lobelia,

Marshmallow, Myrrh, Papaya, Pau D'Arco, *Psyllium, Scullcap, Slippery Elm,* Yellow Dock.

Vitamins: A, B-complex (liquid for quick absorption), C (with bioflavonoids), E, K (deficiency is common).

Minerals: All minerals (liquid), extra herbal calcium, magnesium, chromium, zinc.

Amino Acids: Free-form amino acids (between meals).

Supplements: Linseed Oil, Evening Primrose Oil, or Black Currant Oil; Acidophilus (milk free), Liquid Chlorophyll, Aloe Vera Juice, Glucomannan (before meals); Bentonite, Algin, Fish Oil Lipids, Echinacea Extract; Nutritional Fiber Supplement.

Colon Health

Colon health is essential to overall health. Almost any disease can be improved when the colon is cleaned. A high protein diet promotes bacteria growth and the absorption of toxins into the bloodstream. Intestinal toxemia is the most critical primary cause of many illnesses and diseases.

Herbal Combinations: Blood Purifier, Cleansing, Digestion, General Cleanser, Immune, Liver and Gall Bladder, Lower Bowel, Red Clover.

Regulate Bowels: Comfrey and Pepsin, Cascara Sagrada, General Cleanser, Combination and Lower Bowel Combination.

Single Herbs: Aloe Vera, Alfalfa, Barberry, Buckthorn, Burdock, *Cascara Sagrada, Comfrey,* Dandelion, Fennel, Fenugreek, Ginger, Golden Seal, Kelp, Licorice, Mullein, Myrrh, Pau D'Arco, *Psyllium,* Senna, *Slippery Elm,* Yarrow.

Vitamins: A, B-complex, D.E.

Minerals: Multi-minerals (liquid), calcium and magnesium (balance), selenium, zinc.

Amino Acids: Free-form amino acids.

Supplements: Apple Pectin, Acidophilus, Chlorophyll, Bran Tablets, Flaxseed, Wheat Grass; High Fiber Diet; Algin, Bentonite.

Cystic Fibrosis

Cystic Fibrosis is an inherited disease seen early in infants. Exercise to help keep the lungs healthy and clear of mucus is important in the treatment of cystic fibrosis. Also, because there is a lack of enzymes for digestion, a change in diet is essential to help the healing. The diet should include: Raw fruits and vegetables; steamed vegetables (drink juice), fruit and vegetable juices; raw oils, nuts, seeds, honey, and sprouts; baked potatoes, squash and yams.

Herbal Combinations: Anemia, Glands, Digestion (enzymes), Immune, Lungs.

Single Herbs: Alfalfa, Catnip, Capsicum, *Comfrey, Fennel, Ginger,* Hops, Kelp, Licorice, *Lady's Slipper,*

Lobelia, Marshmallow, Mullein, *Papaya,* Peppermint, Pau D'Arco, Red Clover, *Safflower, Saffron (digest fats),* Scullcap, *Slippery Elm.*

Vitamins: A (every day--builds healthy mucus membranes), C (high amounts daily), E (deficiency is seen).

Minerals: Multi-minerals (liquid), selenium (seen as deficient), zinc.

Amino Acids: L-Cysteine, L-Methionine.

Supplements: Chlorophyll, Glucomannan (won't absorb--keeps colon clean), Evening Primrose Oil, Black Currant Oil.

Cysts

Cysts are usually benign, but can turn cancerous if not taken care of. For treatment of cysts, avoid meat, dairy products and caffeine drinks (caffeine has been linked to fibrocystic disease). Tumors and growths have been eliminated by cleansing inside and using herbs.

Herbal Combinations: Blood Purifier, Bone Combination, Cleansing, General Cleanser, Immune, Lower Bowels, stress.

Single Herbs: Alfalfa, *Burdock,* Cascara Sagrada, *Chaparral,* Hops, Horsetail, Kelp, Lobelia, Mullein, Oatstraw, *Pau D'Arco, Red Clover,* Scullcap, Yellow Dock.

Vitamins: A, B-complex (extra B6, B12), C (with

bioflavonoids), E (helps reduce cysts).

Minerals: Multi-minerals, calcium and magnesium (balance), iron, silicon, sulphur, selenium, zinc.

Amino Acids: Free-form amino acids.

Supplements: High Fiber Diet (low in fat); Evening Primrose Oil (has been shown to reduce cysts); Chlorophyll, Spirulina, Lecithin, Black Ointment.

Depression

Depression is caused by stress, tension, allergies, imbalanced body and hormonal imbalance. It is helpful to avoid additives, preservatives and chemical pollutants. Hypoglycemia can cause depression and can be controlled by a diet that avoids sugar, dairy products, chocolate and caffeine products.

Herbal Combinations: Anemia, Blood Purifier, Bone, Digestion, Immune, Lower Bowels, Nerve and Relaxant, Stress.
Single Herbs: Alfalfa, Black Cohosh, Black Walnut, *Burdock*, Capsicum, Chaparral, Dandelion, Dong Quai, *Ephedra,* Echinacea, Garlic, Ginger, *Ginseng,* Golden Seal, *Gotu Kola*, Hawthorn, Hops, *Ho Shou-Wu,* Lady's Slipper, *Licorice,* Lobelia, Passion Flower, Red Raspberry, Red Clover, Sarsaparilla, Scullcap, St. Johnswort, Watercress, Wood Betony, Yellow Dock.

Vitamins: A, B-complex (with extra B6, B12, folic acid, niacin), C (with bioflavonoids), choline, inositol, pantothenic acid.

Minerals: Multi-minerals, calcium and magnesium (balance), selenium, zinc.

Amino Acids: Free-form amino acids, Tryptophan, Tyrosine, Glutamine, Phenylalanine, Taurine.

Supplements: Bee Pollen, Spirulina, Chlorophyll, Evening Primrose Oil, Black Currant Oil; Brown Rice, Whole Grains, Beans and Lentils, Safflower Oil, Rice Bran Syrup.

Diabetes

Diabetes results when there is a malfunction of the pancreas. This can be a very serious disease, resulting in a loss of vision and a loss of circulation in the legs if it's not corrected.

Herbal Combinations: Blood Purifier, Bone, Lower Bowels, Pancreas and Diabetes, Parasites and Worms, Potassium, Stress.

Single Herbs: *Alfalfa,* Black Walnut, Buchu, *Burdock,* Capsicum, Chaparral, Cornsilk, Dandelion, Echinacea, *Garlic,* Gentian, Ginger, Ginseng, *Golden Seal (acts as insulin),* Hawthorn, Horsetail, Irish Moss, Juniper Berries, Kelp, Licorice, Lobelia, Myrrh, Parsley, Psyllium, Queen of the Meadow, *Red Clover,* Sarsaparilla, *Uva Ursi, Watercress,* Wormwood, Yarrow, *Yellow Dock.*

Vitamins: A, B-complex (extra biotin, inositol and choline), C (with bioflavonoids--1,000 milligrams three times a day), E.

Minerals: Calcium and magnesium (balance), manganese, potassium, zinc (depleted in diabetics).

Amino Acids: Arginine, Taurine, Glutamic Acid, Cysteine, Glycine, Phenylalanine (essential for production of adrenaline).

Supplements: High Fiber Diet, Lecithin, Glucomannan, Chlorophyll, Rice Bran Syrup.

Diarrhea

Diarrhea can stem from parasites, colitis, stress, viruses, chemicals, allergies, and/or food allergies. It is important to watch for dehydration when diarrhea is a problem.

Herbal Combinations: Blood Purifier, Cleansing, Colitis, Digestion, Glands, Lower Bowels, Nerve and Relaxant, Potassium.

Single Herbs: Alfalfa, Bayberry, Capsicum, Comfrey, Chamomile Tea, Dandelion, Garlic, Gentian, Ginger, Golden Seal, Hawthorn, Kelp, Licorice, Lobelia, Myrrh, Oatstraw, *Raspberry (tea),* Red Clover, *Slippery Elm,* White Oak Bark, Wormwood.

Vitamins: A, C (with bioflavonoids).

Minerals: Multi-minerals (they are lost during diarrhea), extra calcium, potassium, zinc.

Supplements: Glucomannan, Acidophilus, Evening Primrose Oil, Charcoal Tablets, Barley Water, Carob

Drink, Blackberry Juice.

Edema

Edema is abnormal fluid retention in the body--resulting in swelling and bloating, which can cause depression. Edema can be caused by allergies to certain foods, salt intake and too much animal products. Bad colon health is considered to be a main cause of edema. It is beneficial to have daily exercise--a walk in fresh air, mini-trampoline.

Herbal Combinations: Bladder and Kidney, Bone Combination, Digestion, Lower Bowels.

Single Herbs: *Alfalfa,* Aloe Vera, *Buchu,* Burdock, Capsicum, Comfrey, *Cornsilk,* Dandelion, Fenugreek, *Garlic,* Ginger, Horsetail, *Hydrangea,* Juniper Berries, Kelp, *Licorice,* Lobelia, Oatstraw, Marshmallow, *Parsley*, Pau D'Arco, Queen of the Meadow, Spirulina, *Uva Ursi,* Watercress, Yarrow.
Vitamins: A, B-complex (with extra B1, B6), C, E.

Minerals: Calcium and magnesium (balance), silicon, sulphur, selenium, zinc.

Amino Acids: L-Taurine.

Supplements: Liquid Chlorophyll, Mullein and Lobelia (together).

Ear Infections

Allergies to dairy products are one cause of ear infections. Grains can also be a cause of ear infections--infants should not be given any grains until after they are one year old. Ear infections have been linked to various types of allergies.

Herbal Combinations: Colds & Flu, Infections, Lower Bowels, Nerve and Relaxant.

Single Herbs: Alfalfa, Black Walnut, Capsicum, *Catnip,* Chamomile, Cornsilk, Dandelion, *Garlic (oil),* Ginger, Gotu Kola, Hawthorn, Hops, Horsetail *Lady's Slipper*, Licorice, Lobelia (relaxer), *Mullein Oil (pain),* Pau D'Arco, Red Clover, Scullcap, Slippery Elm, Valerian, *White Willow, Wood Betony,* Yarrow, Yellow Dock.

Vitamins: A, C (with bioflavonoids), E (liquid--for children or those who have poor digestion).

Minerals: Calcium and magnesium (balance), manganese, zinc.
Amino Acids: Free-form amino acids.

Supplements: Liquid Chlorophyll, Garlic Oil (in ear for infection), Mullein Oil (helps in pain), Raw Goat's Milk, Echinacea Extract, Peppermint Oil.

Epstein-Barr

Epstein-Barr is a low-grade flu-like virus. It is a member of the herpes family and can cause mononucleosis and infections. Symptoms of Epstein-Barr are muscle weakness, and achy, swollen lymph glands. It brings on extreme fatigue, irritability, memory loss, and poor concentration. This virus lowers the immune system.

Herbal Combinations: Blood Purifier, Digestion, Glands, Infection, Immune, Liver, Nerve Relaxant, Stress.

Single Herbs: Aloe Vera, Buchu, Burdock, Capsicum, Comfrey, Cornsilk, Dandelion, *Echinacea (glands),* Garlic, Ginger, Golden Seal, Hawthorn, *Horsetail,* Licorice, *Lobelia,* Myrrh, *Oatstraw,* Pau D'Arco (blood cleanser), Parsley, *Red Clover,* Saffron or Safflower (helps stop aches), *Scullcap,* Watercress, Yellow Dock.

Vitamins: A, B-complex (with extra folic acid, B12), C (with bioflavonoids).

Minerals: Multi-minerals, extra selenium, zinc.

Amino Acids: Free-form amino acids (between meals, extra Lysine, Methionine, Threonine, Valine.
Supplements: Acidophilus, Black Currant Oil, Evening Primrose Oil, Garlic Oil, Golden Seal/Echinacea Extract.

Epilepsy

Epilepsy can result from injuries, scar tissue, food allergies, infections and/or worms. It is caused by electrical disturbances in the nerve cells of the brain. Effective brain circulation and a healthy diet are important. Regular bowel function is essential. (English researchers have shown that extreme amounts of aspartame or Nutra Sweet causes epilepsy).

Herbal Combinations: Blood Cleanser, Digestion, Glands, Heart, Nerve and Relaxant, Lower Bowels.

Single Herbs: Alfalfa, Black Cohosh, Black Walnut (if parasites), Burdock, Capsicum, Dandelion, Echinacea, *Garlic,* Gentian, Ginger, *Gotu Kola,* Hawthorn, *Hops,* Licorice, *Lady's Slipper*, Lobelia, Myrrh, *Passion Flower*, *Pau D'Arco*, Red Clover, *Scullcap, Valerian*, Yellow Dock.

Vitamins: A, B-complex (with extra B6, B12, folic acid, pantothenic acid, pangamic acid), C (with bioflavonoids), D, E.

Minerals: Calcium and magnesium (balance--250 mg.), chromium, manganese, zinc.

Amino Acids: Taurine, Tryptophan, Glutamine (detoxifies ammonia from brain).

Supplements: Black Currant Oil, Green Drinks, Chlorophyll, Acidophilus, Lecithin, Psyllium, Glucomannan, Bee Pollen and Spirulina, Senna Tea, Juice Fasts, Vegetable and Fruit, Rice Bran Syrup.

Eyes

Eye examinations are very important because many diseases can be seen in the eyes by a specialist. Iridology can also determine weakness in the body. Inflammation, sore eyes, cataracts and glaucoma are some conditions of the eyes. Cataracts form when vitamin C, B2, Lysine and Tryptophan are low.

Herbal Combinations: Allergies, Blood Purifier, Digestion, Eye, Heart, Immune, Infection (where infections), Lower Bowels, Stress.

Single Herbs: Aloe Vera, Bayberry, Bilberry, Black Cohosh, Black Walnut, Burdock, *Capsicum,* Chaparral, Comfrey, Echinacea, *Eyebright*, Fenugreek, Garlic, Ginger, Ginseng, *Golden Seal,* Gotu Kola, Grapevine, *Hops*, Ho Shou-Wu, Hawthorn, Kelp, Lady's Slipper, Licorice, *Lobelia,* Mistletoe, Myrrh, Oatstraw, *Passion Flower,* Red Clover, *Scullcap*, St. Johnswort, *Valerian,* White Oak, Wood Betony, Yellow Dock.

Vitamins: A, B-complex (with extra B2, B3, B12), C (with bioflavonoids), E, F.

Minerals: Calcium and magnesium (balance), manganese, selenium, zinc.

Amino Acids: Lysine, Tryptophan, Phenylalanine (protects eyes).

Supplements: Evening Primrose Oil, Black Currant Oil, Chlorophyll.

Fasting

The best protection to the immune system is to fast occasionally and let the body detoxify and renew itself. This cleans the body of built-up toxins, air pollution, and many other poisons we are confronted with constantly.

It can be accomplished by one day each month, three days each month, or two or three times a year.

Herbal Combinations: There are many herbal combinations to support the system while fasting. They can be taken before a fast to prepare the body gradually. You can decide on the combinations that work best for you. Suggested combinations are: Blood Purifier, Chelation, Cleansing, Endurance, Fasting or Dieting, Energy and Fitness, General Cleanser, Glands, Heart and Blood Pressure, Hypoglycemia, Immune, Lower bowels, Nerve and Relaxant, Parasites and Worms.

Single Herbs: Alfalfa, Aloe Vera, Bayberry, Black Walnut, Buchu, Buckthorn, Burdock, Capsicum, *Cascara Sagrada,* Cornsilk, Dandelion, Echinacea, *Garlic,* Ginger, Ginseng, Golden Seal, *Hawthorn,* Horsetail, Juniper Berries, *Kelp, Licorice, Lobelia,* Parsley, *Pau D'Arco,* Psyllium, Queen of the Meadow, *Red Clover,* Rhubarb, Rose Hips, *Slippery Elm,* Uva Ursi, Watercress, Yarrow, Yellow Dock.

Vitamins: Some are helpful in cleansing--like vitamin C (with bioflavonoids).

Minerals: Calcium and magnesium (balance), potassium, liquid minerals.

Amino Acids: Free-form amino acids are very strengthening to the system.

Supplements: Vegetable Broth, Liquid Chlorophyll, Acidophilus, Carrot and Celery Juice, Green Drinks; Lemon Juice and Maple Syrup Cleanse; herbal Teas such as Red Clover Blend and Pau D'Arco.

Fatigue

Fatigue can refer to physical or mental exhaustion. It can be caused by anemia or allergies. A high fat and sugar diet can cause chronic fatigue, as well as poor diet, obesity, infections, hypoglycemia and stress. Alcohol, smoking and caffeine can also be a cause.

Herbal Combinations: Anemia, Blood Purifier, Bone, Candida (cleansing), Digestion, Endurance, Energy and Fitness, General Cleanser, Hypoglycemia, Immune, Lower Bowels, Stress.

Single Herbs: Alfalfa, Black Cohosh, Burdock, Capsicum, Chaparral, Dandelion, *Dong Quai,* Garlic, *Ginseng*, Gentian, Golden Seal, *Gotu Kola,* Hawthorn, Hops, *Ho Shou-Wu, Kelp, Licorice,* Lobelia, Mistletoe, Myrrh, *Red Clover,* Scullcap, St. Johnswort, Valerian, Wood Betony, Wormwood, Yellow dock.

Vitamins: Multi-vitamins, B-complex (extra B6, B12), C (with bioflavonoids), E.

Minerals: Multi-minerals (liquid), extra calcium and magnesium (balance), chromium, iron, potassium, zinc.

Amino Acids: Free-form amino acids (liquid--between meals), Leucine (increases energy).

Supplements: Acidophilus, Chlorophyll, Herbal Teas, Algin, Black Currant Oil or Evening Primrose Oil.

Female Problems

Female problems refer to those such as: Endometriosis, leucorrhea, cysts, tumors, menopause, menstrual problems. Female problems stem from an imbalanced body (nutritional or hormonal imbalance). When the body is cleansed and the diet changed, along with added herbs, vitamins, minerals and special supplements, many problems have cleared up.

Herbal Combinations: These combinations are formulated to clean the body and balance hormones: Blood Purifier, Energy and Fitness, Female Problems, General Cleanser, Glands, Immune, Infections (for infections), Insomnia, Lower Bowels, Menopause, Nerves, Relaxant, Potassium, Premenstrual, Stress.

Single Herbs: Alfalfa, *Black Cohosh*, Black Walnut, Burdock, Capsicum, Chaparral, Cramp bark, Dandelion, *Damiana, Dong Quai, False Unicorn,* Garlic, Gentian, Ginger, Ginseng, Golden Seal, *Gotu Kola,* Hops, Ho Shou-Wu, Hawthorn, Irish Moss, *Kelp, Licorice,* Lobelia, Mistletoe, Myrrh, Red Clover, Red Raspberry, *Sarsaparilla, Saw Palmetto*, Scullcap, *Squaw Vine,* Watercress, Wood Betony, Wormwood, Yellow Dock.

Vitamins: A, B-complex (with extra B5, B6, PABA--substitute for estrogen B12), C (with bioflavonoids), D, E (stimulated estrogen production), choline and inositol (necessary to detoxify estrogen by the liver).

Minerals: Multi-minerals, extra calcium and magnesium (balance), manganese, selenium, silicon, zinc.

Amino Acids: Free-form amino acids (liquid--between meals).

Supplements: Essential fatty acids in the Evening Primrose Oil or Black Currant Oil; Lecithin; exercise and learn to handle stress; Fish Oil Lipids, Spirulina, Chelated Cell Salts.

Food Poisoning

If a chemical or drug poisoning takes place, call the doctor or poison control center. Food poisoning is common during the summer. Salmonella, one of the most common types of food poisoning, can result from eating bad eggs, meat or chicken.

Herbal Combinations: Blood Purifier, Cleansing, Colds and Flu, Digestion, General Cleanser, Lower Bowels, Nerve and Relaxant, Stress.

Single Herbs: Alfalfa, Aloe Vera, Bayberry, Black Walnut, Buckthorn, Burdock, Capsicum, Cascara Sagrada, *Catnip*, Chaparral, Dandelion, Echinacea, Garlic, Gentian, *Ginger*, Ginseng, *Golden Seal,* Hawthorn, Irish Moss, *Kelp,* Licorice, Lobelia, Myrrh, Psyllium, *Red Clover*, Rhubarb, Rosemary, Watercress, Wormwood, Yarrow, Yellow Dock.

Vitamins: A (emulsion--enters system faster), liquid vitamins, C (to help detoxify).

Minerals: Multi-minerals (depleted fast when vomiting), potassium (lost quickly).

Amino Acids: Free-form amino acids (enter system quickly for tissue repair).

Supplements: Acidophilus, Algin, Ipecac (induce vomiting, Charcoal (absorbs toxins); Enemas will help rid toxins faster; Chinese Essential Oils, Golden Seal/Echinacea Extract.

Gallbladder

Common gallbladder ailments are gallstones and infections. An olive oil and lemon juice fast can help dissolve gallstones.

Herbal Combinations: Blood Cleanser, Bone Chelation, Cleansing, Digestion, General Cleanser, Infection, Liver and Gallbladder, Lower Bowels.

Single Herbs: Aloe Vera, Barberry, Black Walnut, Burdock, Capsicum, Catnip, Chaparral, Comfrey, Cramp Bark, *Dandelion,* Echinacea, Fennel, Fenugreek, *Garlic,* Ginger, Golden Seal, Gotu Kola, Hawthorn, Hops, Horsetail, *Hydrangea,* Licorice, Lobelia, Mistletoe, Myrrh, Parsley, Oatstraw, Red Clover, Rosemary, Sarsaparilla, Scullcap, St. Johnswort, White Oak Bark, Wild Yam, Yellow Dock.

Vitamins: A, B-complex (with extra B12, choline and inositol), D, C (with bioflavonoids).

Minerals: Multi-minerals, potassium, zinc.

Supplements: Lecithin, Evening Primrose Oil, Black Currant Oil, flaxseeds, almonds, sesame seeds.

Glands

The lymph glands remove toxins from the body. They are the body's filter system. If the lymph glands are not working properly, the toxins build up in the bloodstream.

Adrenals: Hypoglycemia Combination, Brigham Tea, Licorice, Rose Hips and Capsicum, Ginseng, Vitamin C, B-complex, Calcium and Pantothenic Acid.

Pituitary: Alfalfa, Licorice, Ginseng, Gotu Kola and Ho Shou-Wu.

Thyroid: Glands and Thyroid combinations, Black Walnut, Kelp (for goiter), White Oak Bark.

Female: Female Problems Combination, Black Cohosh, Dong Quai, Damiana, Yellow Dock, Vitamin C, Calcium, Iron.

Male: Prostate and Sex Rejuvenation Combinations, Ginseng, Vitamin A, C, E, Zinc.

Male or Female: Menopause Combination, Ginseng, Golden Seal, Saw Palmetto, Bee Pollen, Lecithin, Vitamin A, B, C, E, Zinc.

Herbal Combinations: Blood Purifier, Endurance, Energy and Fitness, Glands.

Single Herbs: Alfalfa, Barberry, *Black Cohosh,* Black Walnut, Burdock, Capsicum, Dandelion, Dong Quai, *Echinacea,* Garlic, Gentian, *Ginseng,* Golden Seal, Gotu Kola, Hawthorn, Hops, Ho Shou-Wu, *Kelp, Licorice,*

Lobelia and Mullein together, Myrrh, Oregon Grape, Parsley, Pau D'Arco, Red Clover, *Sarsaparilla,* Scullcap, St. Johnswort, Valerian, Watercress, Wood Betony, Wormwood, Yellow Dock, Yucca.

Vitamins: A, B-complex (with extra pantothenic acid), C (with bioflavonoids).

Minerals: Multi-minerals, silicon, zinc.

Amino Acids: Leucine (assists function of the glands), Valine (necessary for glandular function).

Supplements: Evening Primrose Oil, Linseed Oil, Bentonite Cleanse, Black Currant Oil or Evening Primrose Oil, Chelated Cell Salts, Fish Oil Lipids, Golden Seal, Echinacea Extract.

Guillain-Barre Syndrome

Guillain-Barre syndrome is a disease causing muscle weakness and inflammation of nerve roots. It causes motor loss. Guillain-Barre syndrome can start with upper respiratory tract infections, too much sugar products, rabies, swine flu vaccinations, or virus illnesses.

Herbal Combinations: Blood Purifier, Bone Combination, Cleansing, Digestion, General Cleanser, Glands, Immune, Infection, Lungs, Nerve and Relaxant, Pain, Stress.

Single Herbs: Alfalfa, *Aloe Vera*, Black Cohosh, *Black Walnut, Blue Vervain Extract*, Burdock, Capsicum, Chaparral, Cascara Sagrada, *Comfrey, Cornsilk,*

Dandelion, Echinacea, Garlic, Gentian, Ginger, Ginseng, Golden Seal, *Gotu Kola,* Hawthorn, Hops, *Horsetail,* Ho Shou-Wu, Irish Moss, Juniper, Kelp, *Licorice, Lobelia,* Marshmallow, Mistletoe, Myrrh, Parsley, Psyllium, *Queen of the Meadow,* Sarsaparilla, *Scullcap,* Slippery Elm, St. Johnswort, Uva Ursi, *Valerian,* Watercress, *Wood Betony,* Wormwood, Yarrow, Yellow Dock, Yucca.

Vitamins: Multi-vitamins, B-complex (extra pantothenic acid), C (with bioflavonoids).

Minerals: Multi-minerals, extra calcium and magnesium (balance), potassium.

Supplements: Liquid Chlorophyll, Green Drinks, Natural Foods, Algin, Spirulina, Black Currant Oil, Evening Primrose Oil, Fish Oil Lipids, Golden Seal/Echinacea extract.

Hair

Nutritional deficiencies can be one cause of hair loss along with stress, protein deficiency, hormonal imbalance or hereditary reasons. Unhealthy liver can result in hair loss. Constant pull on the hairs from things such as braids, curlers, head bands, pony tails and elastic bands can cause breaks and hair loss. Hair needs to be kept clean--it holds dirt and builds up oil, sweat and hair spray.

Herbal Combinations: Blood Purifier, Bone, Female Problems (balance hormones), Hair-Skin-Nails, Immune, Nerve and Relaxant, Stress, Thyroid.

Single Herbs: *Alfalfa*, Black Cohosh (balance hormones), Blessed Thistle, *Comfrey*, Dulse, *Horsetail*, *Jojoba*, Kelp (rich in minerals), Licorice (helps adrenals), *Oatstraw*, Parsley, Pau D'Arco, Red Clover, Red Raspberry *Rosemary*, *Sage*,, Sarsaparilla, Slippery Elm, Watercress, Wormwood, *Yarrow*.

Vitamins: A, B-complex (extra biotin, PABA, inositol, pantothenic acid--increases hair growth), C, D, K, E; gray hair needs B6 and pantothenic acid.

Minerals: Multi-mineral, extra iron (Dandelion and Yellow dock--an iron deficiency can lead to hair loss), silicon and sulphur (are essential for hair growth), zinc (deficiency can cause hair loss).

Amino Acids: All amino acids are needed (hair is about 98 percent protein), Cysteine (with vitamin C has increased hair growth).

Supplements: Essential Fatty Acids (Evening Primrose oil, Black Currant oil) helps to conserve protein; Lecithin; eat grains, seeds, nuts, fresh fruit and vegetables; Rice Bran Syrup, Chelated Cell Salts, Fish Oil Lipids.

Headaches

Headaches can be caused by stress, tension, constipation, sinusitis, head injury, air pollution, poor circulation and poor respiration. Allergies to MSG, chocolate, caffeine, wheat, sulfites, sugar, dairy products, alcohol, and vinegar can also be causes.

Herbal Combinations: Allergies, Blood Purifier, Candida, Digestion, Glands, Immune, Lower Bowels, Nerve and Relaxant, Pain, Stress.

Single Herbs: Alfalfa, Aloe Vera, Black Cohosh, Black Walnut, Buchu, Buckthorn, Burdock, Capsicum, Cascara Sagrada, *Chamomile,* Chaparral, Cornsilk, Dandelion, Echinacea, Feverfew, Garlic, Ginger, Ginseng, Golden Seal, Hawthorn, *Hops,* Horsetail, Ho Shou-Wu, Licorice, Psyllium, Red Clover, *Scullcap,* St. Johnswort, Uva Ursi, *White Willow, Wood Betony,* Yarrow, Yellow dock, Yucca.

Vitamins: A, B-complex (with extra niacin, B15 and pangamic acid), C (with bioflavonoids), E.

Minerals: Calcium and magnesium (balance), potassium.

Supplements: Lecithin, Algin, Rice Bran Syrup, Black Currant Oil or Evening Primrose Oil, Chinese Essential Oils, Fish Oil Lipids, Golden Seal/Echinacea Extract, Spirulina, Tea Tree Oil.

Heart

Heart attacks are increasing. They are the leading cause of death in the United States. Lack of exercise and diet are common causes of heart attacks. Poor circulation, which creates an overburdened heart, can cause heart attacks as well as toxic bloodstream.

Herbal Combinations: Blood Purifier, Chelation, Digestion, Heart, Potassium.

Single Herbs: Black Cohosh (for slow pulse rate), *Hawthorn (feeds and strengthens heart), Capsicum, (increases pulse rate), Lobelia (slows down heart palpitation), Garlic (lowers blood pressure), Bugleweed (alleviates pain in heart),* Blessed Thistle, Burdock, *Butchers Broom,* Cramp Bark, Dandelion, *Ephedra,* Garlic Ginseng, Gotu Kola, Hops, *Horsetail,* Hawthorn Berries, Kelp, *Lily of the Valley,* Lobelia, Mistletoe, Oatstraw, *Parsley,* Passion Flower, Rose Hips, Saffron, Scullcap, St. Johnswort, Valerian, Wood Betony, Yarrow.

Vitamins: A, B-complex (extra B3, B6, B14, pangamic acid), E (improves oxygen utilization).

Minerals: Calcium and magnesium (balance), copper, chromium, potassium, selenium (protects heart), zinc.

Amino Acids: Carnitine, Taurine, Histidine, Tryptophan, Cystine.

Supplements: Chlorophyll (rebuilds heart), Lecithin (prevents fatty deposits), Capsicum (1 teaspoon in glass of warm water acts as a first aid for heart attacks), Flaxseeds, Black Currant Oil or Evening Primrose Oil, Fish Oil Lipids, Garlic Oil, Glucomannan, Rice Bran Syrup.

Herpes

Herpes is a very contagious disease that spreads until lesions are healed. Herpes I is cold sores. Herpes II is genital lesion. Herpes is a disease caused by a weakened immune system and needs to be kept under control.

Herbal Combinations: Blood Purifier, Bone Combination, Candida, Cleansing, Colitis, Digestion, Immune, Infection, Lower Bowels, Stress.

Single Herbs: *Aloe Vera Gel (external), Black Walnut (extract),* Comfrey, Garlic, *Golden Seal, Myrrh,* Oregon Grape, *Pau D'Arco,* Red Clover, Rosehips, Slippery Elm.

Vitamins: A, B-complex (yeast free), C (with bioflavonoids), E.

Minerals: Calcium and magnesium (balance), selenium, zinc.

Amino Acids: L-Lysine.

Supplements: Acidophilus; Essential Fatty Acids in fish Lipids, Evening Primrose Oil, Black Currant Oil; Lecithin; Garlic Oil, Golden Seal/Echinacea Extracts, Rice Bran Syrup, Spirulina, Tea Tree Oil.

Hiatal Hernia

Hiatal Hernia is a very common ailment. It is estimated that fifty percent of the people over forty have hiatal hernia. Ulcers often accompany hiatal hernia. Allergies are found to be a cause. It is helpful to watch food combining, and to eat small amounts of food at one time.

Herbal Combinations: Blood Purifier, Bone, Cleansing, Colitis, Digestion (enzymes), Glands, Immune, Lower Bowels, Nerve and Relaxant, Ulcers.

Single Herbs: Alfalfa, *Aloe Vera (heals)*, Black Walnut, Burdock, Capsicum, *Comfrey and Pepsin,* Echinacea, Garlic, Ginger, *Golden Seal,* Hawthorn, Hops, Horsetail, Marshmallow, *Papaya,* Red Clover, Scullcap, Slippery Elm, Yellow9w Dock, Yucca.

Vitamins: A, B-complex, C (with bioflavonoids).

Minerals: Multi-minerals, calcium and magnesium (balance), potassium, zinc.

Supplements: Liquid Chlorophyll, Aloe Vera Juice (use combination of Comfrey, Golden Seal, Slippery Elm and Aloe Vera and mix with apple juice and drink slowly), Black Currant Oil or Evening Primrose Oil, Garlic Oil. Glucomannan, Golden Seal/Echinacea Extracts.

High Blood Pressure

High blood pressure is a symptom of an imbalanced system. It can be caused by bad nutrition--too much meat (animal fat is high in cholesterol). It can also be caused by lack of exercise and nervous disorders--people need to learn to relax. Overeating, tobacco, alcohol, and lack of calcium can also contribute to high blood pressure.

Herbal Combinations: Heart and Blood Pressure, Glands, Nerves, Bone Combination, Chelation, Digestion.

Single Herbs: Alfalfa, Aloe Vera, Black Cohosh, Capsicum, Dandelion, Echinacea, *Garlic,* Ginger, Ginseng, Gotu Kola, *Hawthorn Berries, Hops, Lady's*

Slipper, Mistletoe, Parsley, *Passion Flower,* Pau D'Arco, *Scullcap, Valerian,* Yarrow.

Vitamins: C (with bioflavonoids), K, E (start low).

Minerals: Calcium and magnesium (balance), silicon, sodium.

Amino Acids: Carnitine, Glutamine, Tyrosine.

Supplements: Lecithin, Fish Lipids, Increased Fiber, Evening Primrose Oil or Black Currant Oil, drink Red Clover and Pau D'Arco Tea; Juice Fasts; Glucomannan.

Hormone Imbalance

The hormones are the chemical regulators of the body's systems. They need to be balanced and working in harmony to produce the right amount of hormones.

Herbal Combinations: Blood Purifier, bone and Cleansing, Digestion, Energy and Fitness, Endurance, Female, Female Glandular or Male Glandular, Glands, Immune, Lower Bowels, Nerve and Relaxant, Stress.

Single Herbs: Alfalfa (pituitary), Cedar Berries (pancreas), Kelp (thyroid), Ginseng, *Sarsaparilla (male), Dong Quai, Black Cohosh (female),* Buchu, Burdock, Cornsilk, Dandelion, Echinacea, Garlic, Hawthorn, Horsetail, Juniper, Kelp, Lobelia, Parsley, Red Clover.

Vitamins: Multi-vitamins, A, B-complex (with extra B6), C (with bioflavonoids), E.

Minerals: Multi-minerals, calcium and magnesium (balance), zinc.

Supplements: Grain, raw seeds, nuts sprouts, raw vegetables, and fruits help to balance hormones; Black Currant oil or Evening Primrose Oil, Chelated Cell Salts, Fish Oil Lipids, Golden Seal/Echinacea Extracts, Rice Bran Syrup, Spirulina.

Hyperactivity

Symptoms of hyperactivity are lack of concentration, tantrums, can't sit still, clumsy, insomnia, and learning problems. Sugar is a serious cause of hyperactivity and allergies are suspected to be a cause also. Metal poisoning, and food coloring, flavorings and additives can contribute to hyperactivity.

Herbal Combinations: Allergies, Bone, Cleansing, Glands, Immune, Stress.
Single Herbs: Alfalfa, Black Walnut, Burdock, Catnip, Chaparral, Chickweed, Dandelion, Echinacea, Golden Seal, *Gotu Kola, Hops, Lady's Slipper, Lobelia,* Red Clover, *Scullcap, Wood Betony,* Yellow Dock, Yucca.

Vitamins: A, B-complex (extra B5, B6, and niacin), C (with bioflavonoids).

Minerals: Calcium and magnesium (balance).

Amino Acids: L-Cysteine, Tryptophan (relaxing).

Supplements: Frequent Healthy Snacks, Rice Bran Syrup, Black Currant Oil or Evening Primrose Oil, Spirulina.

Hyperthyroid

Hyperthyroid is an overactive thyroid. Hypothyroid is an underactive thyroid, causing fatigue and overweight. All the glands need to work together, and when the pituitary, parathyroid and six glands become disturbed it can cause problems. There are many diseases that stem from hyperthyroid. A thyroid test, by Broda Barnes, consists of the following: Test before rising in the morning. Put thermometer in the arm pit for fifteen minutes before rising, lie still. It if read 97.6 degrees or under it could indicate underactive thyroid. Test three days in a row.

Herbal Combinations: Blood Purifier, Bone Combinations, Cleansing, Digestion, Glands, Immune, Stress.

Single Herbs: *Alfalfa,* Bayberry, blue cohosh, black Walnut, *Burdock,* Capsicum, Chaparral, Dandelion, Echinacea, Garlic, Ginger, Ginseng, Golden Seal, *Gotu Kola,* Hawthorn, *Hops,* Ho Shou-Wu, *Kelp,* Ladys' Slipper, *Licorice,* Lobelia, Mistletoe, Parsley, Sarsaparilla, Scullcap, Valerian, Wood Betony, Yellow Dock, Yucca.

Vitamins: A, B-complex (with extra B2, B12), C (with bioflavonoids), E.

Minerals: Multi-minerals, zinc.

Amino Acids: Tryptophan.

Supplements: Lecithin, Black Currant Oil or Evening

Primrose oil, Fish Oil Lipids, Golden Seal/Echinacea Extract.

Hypoglycemia

Hypoglycemia is also referred to as low blood sugar. It is very common in our society which consumes a high amount of sugar products. Food allergies are also found to be linked with hypoglycemia.

Herbal Combinations: Allergies, Bone, Cleansing, Digestion, Endurance, Glands, Hypoglycemia, Immune, Nerves and Relaxant, Pancreas and Diabetes.

Single Herbs: *Alfalfa*, Black Cohosh, Capsicum, *Dandelion,* Garlic, Ginger, *Hawthorn*, Juniper Berries, *Kelp*, Lady's Slipper, *Licorice,* Lobelia, Parsley, *Safflower, Saffron,* Scullcap, Uva Ursi.

Vitamins: B-complex (with extra B1, B3, B5, B6, B12, pantothenic acid), C (with bioflavonoids--helps panic attacks), E.

Supplements: Bee Pollen, Chlorophyll, Green Drinks, Royal Jelly, Lecithin, Spirulina, Wheat Grass, Garlic Oil, Fish Oil Lipids, Rice Bran Syrup, Stevia.

Immune System

A low immune system is indicated by frequent colds, viruses and infections. A low immune system can manifest itself as fatigue, irritability and general susceptibility to disease and infections.

Herbal Combinations: Blood Purifier, Bone Combination, Candida, Cleansing, Digestion, General Cleanser, Glands, Immune, Lower Bowels, Nerves and Relaxant.

Single Herbs: Alfalfa, Burdock, Capsicum, *Chaparral,* Comfrey, *Echinacea, Garlic,* Juniper Berries, Kelp, Lobelia, Mullein, Parsley, *Pau D'Arco,* Red Clover, Sarsaparilla, Watercress.

Vitamins: A, B-complex, C (with bioflavonoids), E.

Minerals: Multi-mineral, calcium and magnesium (balance), potassium, selenium, zinc.

Amino Acids: All are essential for a healthy immune system, extra Cysteine, Methione, Lysine, Ornithine, Taurine, Tryptophan, Phenylalanine, Arginine (supports the immune system).

Supplements: Acidophilus, Evening Primrose Oil, Black Currant Oil, Fish Oil Lipids, Spirulina.

Impotence

Frigidity and impotence can develop because of mental and physical fatigue and stress. Being under constant pressure can lead to impotence. Internal cleansing with herbs and juice fasts can be beneficial by balancing body chemistry.

Herbal Combinations: Blood Purifier, Bone #3, Cleansing, Digestion, Energy and Fitness, Endurance, General Cleanser, Glands, Glandulars, Immune, Lower Bowels, Stress.

Single Herbs: Alfalfa, *Blessed Thistle,* Cramp Bark, Damiana, Echinacea, False Unicorn, *Ginseng,* Gotu Kola, *Ho Shou-Wu,* Kelp, Sarsaparilla, *Saw Palmetto.*

Vitamins: A, B-complex (with extra B3, B4, B6, B12, folic acid and PABA), C (with bioflavonoids), E.

Minerals: Multi-minerals, zinc.

Amino Acids: L-Tyrosine, L-Phenylalanine.

Supplements: Bee Pollen, Lecithin, Fish Oil Lipids, Evening Primrose Oil and Black Currant Oil.

Indigestion

Heartburn, gas and a sluggish feeling can be indications of poor digestion. A common cause of poor digestion is a lack of digestive enzymes. Here is a test to determine if hydrochloric acid is necessary: Take a tablespoon of apple cider vinegar or fresh lemon juice with water. If symptoms are better, then H.C.L. is needed. If the symptoms are worse then H.C.L. is not needed, but here is probably a need for digestive enzymes.

Herbal Combinations: Blood Purifier, Digestion, Liver.

Single Herbs: *Alfalfa, Aloe Vera,* Buchu, Capsicum, *Comfrey,* Cornsilk, Cramp Bark, Dandelion, *Fennel, Garlic,* Gentian, *Ginger,* Ginseng, Gotu Kola, Hawthorn, Hops, Lobelia, Oregon Grape, *Papaya, Parsley,* Peppermint, Scullcap, *Slippery Elm,* Valerian, Wood Betony, Yarrow.

Vitamins: A, B-complex (with extra B1, B3).

Minerals: Multi-minerals, zinc.

Amino Acids: Lysine, Threonine (helps in assimilation of nutrients).

Supplements: Glucomannan, Calcium Combination (helps indigestion), Acidophilus, Aloe Vera Juice; food combining is vital--do not eat meat and starch at the same meal, or vegetables and fruits at the same time; Garlic Oil, Peppermint Oil.

Infertility

Infertility is becoming increasingly more common. The female may have blocked tubes, ovulation problems, hormonal imbalance, weak uterus or nutritional deficiencies which can all cause infertility. The male may have a low sperm count, immature sperm incapable of fertilization or nutritional problems causing infertility.

Herbal Combinations: Anemia, Blood Purifier, Bone Combination, Candida, Cleansing, Digestion, Female, General Cleanser, Glands, Glandular, Immune, Lower Bowels, Nerve and Relaxant, Stress.

Single Herbs: Alfalfa, Chickweed, *Damiana,* Dandelion, *Dong Quai (women),* Echinacea, False Unicorn (strengthens uterus), *Ginseng (men),* Kelp, Licorice, Oatstraw, Pau D'Arco, Red Clover, Red Raspberry, *Sarsaparilla (stimulates progesterone), Saw Palmetto.*

Vitamins: A, B-complex (with extra B6 and pantothenic acid), C (with bioflavonoids), D, E (fertility vitamin).

Minerals: Multi-minerals, iron (Yellow dock), Iodine (Kelp), Manganese, Selenium, Zinc.

Amino Acids: Arginine (increases sperm), Carnitine, Tryptophan.

Supplements: Chlorophyll, Green Drinks; Essential fatty acids in Evening Primrose Oil, Black Currant Oil or Fish Oil Lipids.

Insomnia

Anxiety, distress, pain and nervous exhaustion can cause insomnia. It is necessary to slow down the pace of living. Exercise and fresh air can help, as well as a change of diet--which has a positive effect on the nervous system.

Herbal Combinations: Blood Purifier, Bone, Cleansing, Digestion, General Cleansers, Glands (sometimes helps), Insomnia, Liver (helps), Lower Bowels, Stress.

Single Herbs: Catnip, *Chamomile (tea), Hops, Lady's Slipper (extract), Lobelia, Passion Flower, Scullcap,* Valerian, Wood Betony.

Vitamins: Multi-vitamins, extra B-complex (good for nerves).

Minerals: Calcium and magnesium (balance).

Amino Acids: L-Tryptophan (induces sleep), Valine.

Supplements: Lecithin.

Laryngitis

Laryngitis is the irritation of the larynx or voice box. It can be caused by cold, allergies, emotional stress or infection.

Herbal Combinations: Allergies, Blood Purifier, Infections.

Single Herbs: Echinacea, Ginger, Garlic, *Golden Seal (infections), Licorice and Slippery Elm (hoarseness and coughs), Lobelia Extract (on tongue).*

Vitamins: A, C (with bioflavonoids).

Minerals: Multi-minerals, selenium, zinc.

Supplements: Chinese oils (on tongue), Aloe Vera Juice, Licorice Lozenges, Black Currant Oil or Evening Primrose Oil, Garlic Oil, Golden Seal/Echinacea Extract.

Liver

Hepatitis, alcoholism, viral hepatitis, chronic inflammation and malnutrition can cause liver malfunction. Improper liver function can result in hardening of liver cells and scarred tissues.

Herbal Combinations: Kidney, Liver and Gallbladder, General cleanser, Lower Bowels.

Single Herbs: Alfalfa, Aloe Vera, Barberry, *Burdock, Beet Powder,* Capsicum, Cascara Sagrada, Chaparral, *Dandelion,* Garlic, Golden Seal, Gravel Root, Hops, Horsetail, Kelp, Lobelia, Parsley, *Pau D'Arco, Red Clover*, Rose Hips, Uva Ursi, White Oak, Wood Betony, Yarrow, Yellow Dock.

Vitamins: A, D, B-complex (extra choline), E, K (alfalfa).

Minerals: Calcium and magnesium (balance), zinc.

Amino Acids: Methionine, Cysteine, Asparagine (supports liver function).

Supplements: Chlorophyll, Lecithin, Bentonite Cleanse, Black Currant Oil or Evening Primrose Oil, Fresh Lemon and Pure Water, Fish Oil Lipids, Garlic Oil, Glucomannan, Golden Seal/Echinacea Extract.

Lupus

Lupus is related to arthritis. It is a chronic inflammatory disease which affects many organs. It is suspected that a virus affects the immune system and causes the body to attack itself. Lupus affects the skin. It is beneficial to avoid the nightshade family (tomatoes, potatoes, peppers and eggplant).

Herbal Combinations: Arthritis, Blood Purifier, Bone, Chelation, Cleansing, Digestion, General cleanser, Immune, Lower Bowels, Nerve and Relaxant, Potassium.

Single Herbs: *Aloe Vera,* Black Walnut, *Burdock,* Capsicum, Chaparral, *Comfrey,* Dandelion, *Devil's Claw,* Echinacea, Eyebright, Fenugreek, *Garlic,* Ginger, Golden Seal, Hawthorn, Licorice, Lobelia, Myrrh, Oatstraw, Oregon Grape, *Pau D'Arco, Red Clover,* Sarsaparilla, White Oak, Yellow Dock, *Yucca,* Watercress.

Vitamins: A, B-complex with PABA, C (with bioflavonoids), D.

Minerals: Calcium and magnesium (balance), manganese, zinc.

Amino Acids: L-Cysteine, L-Methionine.

Supplements: Chlorophyll, Acidophilus, Carrot and Celery Juice, Black Currant Oil, Chelated Cell Salts, Chinese Essential Oils (externally for pain), Evening Primrose Oil, Fish Oil Lipids, Garlic Oil, Instant Vitamins, Nutritional Fiber, Spirulina, Tea Tree Oil.

Lymphatic System

The lymphatic system protects against infections. It functions to neutralize and eliminate any poisons or infectious microbes. A sluggish lymphatic system can result in retention of waste materials which could lead to degenerative diseases.

Herbal Combinations: Blood Purifier, General Cleanser, Immune, Infections (swollen glands).

Single Herbs: *Burdock,* Chaparral, *Echinacea,* Golden Seal, *Mullein,* Myrrh, *Lobelia, Pau D'Arco, Red Clover,* Yarrow, Yellow Dock.

Vitamins: A, B-complex (with extra B6), E.

Minerals: Multi-minerals, extra selenium, zinc.

Amino Acids: Phenylalanine, Tyrosine, Cysteine (neutralizes toxins), Tryptophan (cleans blood), Lysine.

Supplements: Walking fast in fresh air (fresh air breathing), exercise on mini-trampoline; Algin, Bentonite Cleanse, Black Currant Oil, Chelated Cell Salts, Evening Primrose Oil, Fish Oil Lipids, Golden Seal/Echinacea Extract, Lecithin, Spirulina.

Meningitis

Meningitis is inflammation of the brain. It is a very serious condition. Symptoms are high fever, stiff neck, chills, nausea and vomiting. It is caused by a bacteria, fungus or virus.

Herbal Combinations: Blood Purifier, Bone Combination, General Cleanser, glands, Immune Infections, Lower Bowels, Nerves and Relaxant, Potassium.

Single Herbs: Aloe Vera, Black Cohosh, *Black Walnut, Buckthorn, Burdock,* Buchu, *Capsicum, Cascara Sagrada,* Catnip, Comfrey, Cornsilk, Dandelion, Fenugreek, Golden Seal, *Gotu Kola, Hawthorn, Hops,* Horsetail, Ho Shou-Wu, *Lady's Slipper,* Licorice,

Lobelia, Myrrh, Oatstraw, Psyllium, Red Clover, Rose Hips, *Scullcap,* White Oak.

Vitamins: A, B (with pantothenic acid).

Minerals: Multi-minerals (vomiting and fever lead to mineral loss), zinc.

Amino Acids: Glutamine, Leucine, Lysine, Methionine, Threonine.

Supplements: Chlorophyll, lots of liquids, enemas, will help bring fever down; Algin, B-complex with Vitamin C and Bioflavonoids, Black Currant Oil, Chelated Cell Salts, Fish Oil Lipids, Golden Seal, Echinacea Extract, Spirulina.

Ménière's Syndrome

Ménière's Syndrome is an inner ear disease. Symptoms are tinnitus, vertigo, nausea, vomiting and possible hearing problems. It can be beneficial to avoid excess meat, dairy products, caffeine drinks and salt.

Herbal Combinations: Blood Cleanser, Hypoglycemia, Glands, Lower Bowels, Nerve and Relaxant.

Single Herbs: Black Cohosh, Black Walnut, Buchu, *Burdock,* Capsicum, Chickweed, Cornsilk, Dandelion, Echinacea, *Garlic,* Ginger, Ginseng, *Gotu Kola, Hawthorn, Hops, Lady's Slipper, Licorice,* Lobelia, Mistletoe, Oregon Grape, Parsley, Queen of the meadow, *Red Clover,* Sarsaparilla, Scullcap, St. Johnswort, Uva Ursi, Wood Betony, Yarrow, Yellow Dock, Yucca, Watercress.

Vitamins: A, B-complex (high doses--extra B1, B2, and niacin), C (with bioflavonoids), E.

Minerals: Calcium and magnesium (balance), manganese, zinc.

Amino Acids: Valine, Glutamine, Tyrosine, Taurine.

Supplements: Bee Pollen, Ginseng Extract, Evening Primrose Oil, Black Currant Oil, Fish Oil Lipids, Hypoglycemia Diet.

Mononucleosis

Fatigue, fever, sore throat and swollen glands are common symptoms for mononucleosis. It is very infectious and is connected to the Epstein-Barr virus. It causes fatigue, flu-like symptoms and muscle pain.

Herbal Combinations: Bladder and Kidneys, Blood Purifier, Bone Combination, Cleansing, Glands, Immune, Infection, Stress.

Single Herbs: Alfalfa, Black Walnut, Buchu, Burdock, Capsicum, Chaparral, Cornsilk, Dandelion, *Echinacea,* Ginger, Golden Seal, *Hawthorn, Hops, Horsetail,* Juniper Berries, Licorice, *Lobelia,* Parsley, *Pau D'Arco, Red Clover,* Uva Ursi, Watercress, Yarrow, Yellow Dock.

Vitamins: A, B-complex (extra B12), E.

Minerals: Calcium and magnesium (balance), potassium, selenium, zinc.

Amino Acids: Free-form amino acids (between meals), extra Leucine, Lysine, Methionine, Threonine and Valine.

Supplements: Acidophilus, Liquid Chlorophyll, Evening Primrose Oil, Black Currant Oil and Fish Oil Lipids.

Mucus

Mucus is a thick fluid which is necessary to lubricate and protect the surface of the mucus membranes. The problem develops when excess mucus accumulates and clogs the system--which causes germs and diseases to invade the body.

Herbal Combinations: Allergy, General Cleanser, Lungs, Digestion, Lower Bowels, Potassium.
Single Herbs: *Comfrey and Pepsin (together),* Aloe Vera, Buchu, Buckthorn, Burdock, Capsicum, Cascara Sagrada, *Comfrey,* Cornsilk, Dandelion, *Echinacea, Fenugreek, Garlic,* Ginger, *Golden Seal,* Hawthorn, *Horsetail,* Licorice, *Lobelia, Marshmallow, Mullein,* Myrrh, Oatstraw, Psyllium, Red Clover, *Slippery Elm,* Yarrow, Yellow Dock.

Vitamins: A, C (with bioflavonoids), E.

Minerals: Multi-minerals (for healthy mucus membranes), potassium, selenium, zinc.

Amino Acids: Cysteine, Taurine, Tryptophan, Cysteine, Glycine, Glumatic Acid and Lysine (sulphur amino acid to destroy free radicals).

Supplements: Juice Fasting; eliminate dairy products, white sugar, white flour and meat; Liquid Chlorophyll.

Multiple Sclerosis

Multiple Sclerosis ia a nervous system disease. It is progressive, degenerative, and affects coordination and vision. It causes numbness and loss of bladder control. Emotional problems, stress and poor nutrition make multiple sclerosis worse.

Herbal Combinations: Digestion, Immune, Nerve and Relaxant, Stress.

Single Herbs: Black Walnut, Burdock, Capsicum, Dandelion, Echinacea, *Garlic*, Gentian, Ginger, *Hawthorn, Hops, Horsetail,* Irish Moss, *Kelp, Lady's Slipper, Licorice, Lobelia,* Marshmallow, Myrrh, Oregon Grape, *Safflower, Saffron, Scullcap,* Valerian, Yellow Dock.

Vitamins: A, B-complex (extra B6, B12, B15), C (with bioflavonoids), D, E.

Minerals: Multi-minerals calcium and magnesium (balance), potassium, phosphorus, manganese (aids in neuromuscular control), selenium, sulphur, zinc.

Amino Acids: Cysteine, Cystine, Leucine, Methionine, Phenylalanine, Tyrosine, Taurine, (Used with A and E-- thought to be very important).

Supplements: Acidophilus, Lecithin, Chlorophyll, Evening Primrose Oil, Black Currant Oil, Fish Oil

Lipids, Rice Bran Syrup.

Muscular Dystrophy

Muscular dystrophy is a disease of the striated muscles which gradually shrivel and weaken. There is about 50% loss of muscle tissue before disease is apparent. It strikes chiefly young children and teenagers. It affects muscles of the trunk of the body. Since inactivity causes constipation it creates a build up of toxins.

Herbal Combinations: Blood Purifier, Bone Combinations, Cleansing, Digestion, General Cleanser, Glands, Immune, Lower Bowels, Pain, Potassium.

Single Herbs: Alfalfa, Aloe Vera, Black Cohosh, Blue Cohosh, *Blue Vervain,* Boneset, Buchu, Burdock, Capsicum, *Comfrey,* Dandelion, *Devil's Claw,* Echinacea, Garlic, Ginseng, Gotu Kola, Hawthorn, Hops, *Horsetail,* Juniper, *Kelp, Lady's Slipper, Licorice, Lobelia,* Mullein, Papaya/Mint, Parsley, Red Clover, Red Raspberry, Saffron, Safflower, Sarsaparilla, *Scullcap, Slippery Elm,* Uva Ursi, Wild Yam, Wood Betony, Yellow Dock.

Vitamins: A, B-complex (extra B1, B12, biotin, niacin, pantothenic acid), E.

Minerals: Calcium and magnesium (balance), potassium (tones muscles), copper, manganese (strengthens coordination).

Amino Acids: Tyrosine, Carnitine (muscle health),

Taurine (feeds muscles and nerves).

Supplements: Evening Primrose Oil, Black Currant Oil, Fish Oil Lipids, Liquid Chlorophyll, Lecithin; keep the bowels clean; natural food is essential--a weak body causes further problems.

Myasthenia Gravis

Myasthenia Gravis causes fatigue, and muscle and skeletal weakness. Emotional stress and infections make it worse. It is a nerve disease which is becoming very common. The nightshade family contains solinase which interferes with the neurotransmitter acetylcholine. Tobacco, white potatoes, tomatoes, peppers and eggplant are some of the nightshade family.

Herbal Combinations: Allergies, Blood Purifier, Bone, Candida, Cleansing, Digestion, Glands, Immune, Lower Bowels, Stress.

Single Herbs: Alfalfa, *Black Cohosh,* Buchu, Burdock, Cornsilk, Dandelion, Echinacea, Garlic Gentian, Ginger, *Gotu Kola,* Hawthorn, *Hops,* Horsetail, Ho Shou-Wu, Kelp, *Lady's Slipper, Licorice, Lobelia,* Parsley, Passion Flower, *Red Clover,* Rosemary, *Scullcap,* St. Johnswort, Valerian, Wood Betony, Yarrow, *Yellow Dock, Yucca.*

Vitamins: A, B-complex (with extra choline, pantothenic acid), C with bioflavonoids).

Minerals: Calcium, manganese (aids in neuromuscular control).

Amino Acids: Valine (muscular coordination), Lysine (builds muscles), methionine (calms nerves), Glycine/Sevine (protects fatty sheaths surrounding nerve fibers), Tyrosine (muscle development).

Supplements: Rice Bran Syrup, Chlorophyll.

Nausea

Morning sickness, flu, food poisoning, emotional upsets or bacterial infections can cause upset stomach and nausea. It is necessary to clean the body to eliminate toxins that can cause nausea in pregnancy.

Herbal Combinations: Anemia, Blood Purifier, Bone, Colds & Flu, Cleansing, Digestion, General Cleanser, Glands, Liver, Lower Bowels, Nerve and Relaxant, Potassium, Stress.

Single Herbs: *Alfalfa,* Catnip, *Fennel,* Fenugreek, *Ginger, Golden Seal, Hops, Kelp,* Lobelia Extract (small doses), *Papaya, Peppermint,* Red Clover, *Red Raspberry,* Scullcap, Wild Yam.

Vitamins: B-complex, C (with bioflavonoids), K and C (together--Alfalfa contains vitamin K, Rose Hips contains vitamin C),

Minerals: Calcium and magnesium (low magnesium can cause nausea), potassium.

Amino Acids: Methionine (aids toxemia in pregnancy to prevent nausea).

Supplements: Alfalfa Mint Tea, Chlorophyll, Alfalfa, Dandelion and Yellow Dock (together); Green Drinks, Lemon and Water.

Nervous Disorders

Nervous disorder diseases are becoming more common. In this condition, the nervous system and spinal cord are affected. Stress, heavy metal poisoning, air pollution and diet can affect the nervous system.

Herbal Combinations: Blood Purifier, Bone Combination, Digestion, Cleansing, Glands, Nerve and Relaxant, Lower Bowels, Potassium, Stress.

Single Herbs: Alfalfa, Aloe Vera, *Black Cohosh,* Black Walnut, *Blue Vervain,* Buchu, Burdock, *Catnip,* Capsicum, Cascara Sagrada, *Chamomile,* Dandelion, Echinacea, Garlic, Gentian, Ginger, Hawthorn, *Hops,* Horsetail, Juniper, Kelp, *Lady's Slipper,* Licorice, *Lobelia Extract,* Parsley, *Passion Flower,* Psyllium, Red Clover, *Scullcap,* Uva Ursi, Valerian, Yellow Dock.

Vitamins: A, B-complex (extra B5 and B12), C (with bioflavonoids).

Minerals: Multi-minerals, extra calcium and magnesium, zinc.

Amino Acids: Valine, Methionine (calms nerves), Tryptophan (soothes nerves).

Supplements: Evening Primrose Oil, Black Currant Oil, Fish Oil Lipids, Lecithin.

Obesity

It is essential to eliminate fats and sweets that are rich in calories for treatment of obesity. Allergies are often connected with overweight. For treatment of obesity, eating habits need to be changed--work with a rotation diet, a cleansing diet and use juice fasts frequently. Exercise is very important.

Herbal Combinations: Blood Purifier, Cleansing, digestion, Fasting and Dieting, Glands, Glandular, Lower Bowels, Stress, Weight Control Aids.

Single Herbs: *Alfalfa,* Black Cohosh, Black Walnut, Burdock, Capsicum, Cascara Sagrada, *Chickweed,* Comfrey, Dandelion, Echinacea, Gentian, Gotu Kola, *Fennel, Hawthorn,* Hops, *Horsetail,* Ho Shou Wu, *Kelp, Lady's Slipper,* Licorice, Lobelia, Marshmallow, Papaya, Parsley, Passion Flower, *Psyllium, Safflower, Saffron,* Sarsaparilla, Scullcap, Senna, *Slippery Elm,* Watercress, Yellow Dock.

Vitamins: Multi-vitamins, B-complex Extra B6, B12, pantothenic acid, choline and inositol--breaks down fat), C (with bioflavonoids), E.

Minerals: Multi-minerals, calcium and magnesium (balance), potassium, zinc.

Amino Acids: Carnitine, Phenylalanine, Ornithine, Arginine, Lysine, Leucine (regulates digestion and metabolism).

Supplements: Bee Pollen, Flaxseed, Evening Primrose Oil, Glucomannan, Apple Cider Vinegar, Lecithin,

Vitamin B6, Kelp, Spirulina, Rice Bran Syrup.

Osteoporosis

Osteoporosis is a bone disease caused by a malabsorption of calcium into the bones. It can be hereditary or caused by alcohol, smoking, birth control pills, high sugar and/or high phosphorus intake. Some heavy toxic metals can prevent absorption of minerals and calcium--hydrochloric acid is necessary for calcium absorption. High meat diets, phosphate drinks, and some drugs leach out calcium.

Herbal Combinations: Bone, Digestion, Glands.

Single Herbs: *Alfalfa,* Black Walnut, Burdock, Capsicum, Catnip, Chaparral, *Comfrey,* Dandelion, Echinacea, Garlic, Ginger, Ginseng, Golden Seal, Hawthorn, *Horsetail* , Irish Moss, *Kelp*, Licorice, Lobelia, Marshmallow, *Oatstraw,* Papaya, Plantain, *Red Clover,* Sarsaparilla, *Slippery Elm.*

Vitamins: A, B-complex (extra B6, B12), C (with bioflavonoids), De, E.

Minerals: Magnesium (to balance calcium--too much calcium blocks the absorption of magnesium), potassium, silicon, sulphur.

Amino Acids: Lysine (with vitamin C--helps in assimilation of calcium), Leucine (regulates metabolism and digestion).

Supplements: Molasses, Fish Liver Oils, Fish Oil Lipids, Evening Primrose Oil.

Parasites and Worms

Parasites and worms are suspected to be involved in diseases such as cancer, lupus, sinus trouble and arthritis was well as other diseases. When there are sufficient amounts of healthy bile (hydrochloric acid), the parasites, worms, larva and eggs are neutralized and evacuated rapidly.

Herbal Combinations: Blood Purifier, Digestion, Immune, Liver, Lower Bowels, Parasites and Worms, Potassium.

Single Herbs: Alfalfa, Aloe Vera, *Black Walnut* and *Burdock (equal parts for purging out parasites and worms),* Buchu, Catnip, *Chaparral,* Cornsilk, Echinacea, Garlic, Hops, Horsetail, Gotu Kola, *Kelp,* Lady's Slipper, Lobelia, Papaya, Parsley, Pau D'Arco, Peppermint, *Psyllium,* Queen of the Meadow, Red Clover, Senna, St. Johnswort, Uva Ursi, Wood Betony, Wormwood, Yarrow, Yellow Dock.

Vitamins: A, B-complex, C.

Minerals: Multi-minerals (discourages parasites and worms), selenium, zinc.

Amino Acid: Leucine, Methionine, Threonine, Arginine (detoxifies blood).

Supplements: Pumpkin Seeds (grind and put on food), Chlorophyll (clean blood), Algin, Bentonite, Chelated Cell Salts, Garlic Oil, Glucomannan, Golden Seal/Echinacea Extract, Spirulina.

Parkinson's Disease

Parkinson's disease is a central nervous system disease causing shaking, stiffness and memory loss. Heavy metals are toxic to the central nervous system-- such as aluminum-- and are suspected as being one cause of Parkinson's disease. Exercise and proper diet can slow down its progress.

Herbal Combinations: Blood Purifier, Bone, Chelation, digestion, Cleansing, Liver and Gall Bladder, Lower Bowels, Nerve and Relaxant, Stress.

Single Herbs: Alfalfa, *Black Cohosh*, Black Walnut, Burdock, Capsicum, Chaparral, Comfrey, Echinacea, Garlic, Ginger, Ginseng, Golden Seal, *Gotu Kola, Hawthorn, Hops,* Horsetail, Ho Shou-Wu, Kelp, *Lady's Slipper, Lobelia,* Mistletoe, *Passion Flower, Red Clover, Scullcap,* St. Johnswort, *Valerian, Wood Betony,* Yellow Dock.

Vitamins: A, B-complex (*extra B6, B12, niacin), C (with bioflavonoids), E.

Minerals: Multi-minerals, selenium, zinc.

Amino Acids: Tryptophan, Tyrosine, Glutamic Acid, Valine, Phenylalanine.

Supplements: Algin, Chlorophyll, Lecithin; a high fiber diet--grains, seeds, and nuts.

Premenstrual Tension

Menstrual problems can cause cramps, depression, breast swelling, water retention, insomnia, fatigue, nervousness and personality changes. Allergies to foods such as chocolate and caffeine can cause symptoms to worsen. Exercise is very beneficial.

Herbal Combinations: Anemia, Bone, Digestion, Female, Glands, Glandular, Nerve and Relaxant, Premenstrual.

Single Herbs: Alfalfa, *Black Cohosh, Blessed Thistle,* Burdock, Chamomile; *Damiana, Dong Quai, False Unicorn,* Gentian, Gotu Kola, *Hawthorn,* Hops, Horsetail, *Kelp,* Licorice, *Lobelia,* Parsley, *Red Clover, Red Raspberry, Sarsaparilla,* Scullcap, *Squaw vine, Saw Palmetto,* Valerian, Wood Betony, Yellow Dock.

Vitamins: A, B-complex (extra B6, B12, pantothenic acid), C (with bioflavonoids), E.

Minerals: Multi-minerals, extra iron (Dandelion and Yellow Dock), potassium, magnesium (helps calcium absorption, works with B6), silicon (horsetail).

Amino Acids: Tyrosine, Phenylalanine.

Supplements: Evening Primrose Oil, Black Currant Oil, Fish Oil Lipids; Magnesium-rich foods such as beans, bran and dark green vegetables; Spirulina, Molasses, Chelated Cell Salts, Chlorophyll, Spirulina.

Prostate

Urinary problems and painful and urgent urination are common prostate disorders. Prostate cancer is increasing. Alcohol, caffeine, and nicotine have negative effects on the prostate. Hot sitz baths are beneficial.

Herbal Combinations: Blood Purifier, Chelation, General Cleanser, Glands, Glandular, Immune, Infections, Kidney, Lower Bowels, Pain, Prostate.

Single Herbs: *Alfalfa,* Black Cohosh, Black Walnut, Blessed Thistle, *Buchu,* Burdock, Chaparral, Capsicum, *Comfrey, Cornsilk, Damiana,* Dandelion, Echinacea, False Unicorn, Garlic, Ginger, Ginseng, Golden Seal, Hawthorn, Hops, Horsetail, *Juniper Berries,* Kelp, Lady's Slipper, Marshmallow, *Parsley,* Pau D'Arco, Red Clover, Red Raspberry, Saw Palmetto, Scullcap, Slippery Elm, St. Johnswort, *Uva Ursi,* Wood Betony, Yarrow, Yellow Dock.

Vitamins: A, B-complex (extra B6), E.

Minerals: Multi-minerals, magnesium, potassium, silicon, zinc.

Amino Acids: Methionine, Arginine, Cystine, Histidine (with B6 and niacin).

Supplements: Bee Pollen, Fish Oil Lipids, Chlorophyll, Lecithin, Pumpkin Seeds.

Retardation

Retardation causes autism and learning disabilities in children. Check for allergies and heavy metal accumulation.

Herbal Combinations: Allergies, Blood Purifier, Immune Parasites and Worms, Stress.

Single Herbs: *Alfalfa,* Black Walnut, Dandelion, Echinacea, Garlic, *Gotu Kola,* Hawthorn, *Hops, Lady's Slipper,* Licorice, Lobelia, *Red Clover, Scullcap,* Wood Betony, Yellow Dock.

Vitamins: B-complex (extra B6, niacin, pantothenic acid), liquid vitamins (for children--easier to absorb), C (with bioflavonoids), E.

Minerals: Magnesium, zinc (liquid is best).

Amino Acids: Glutamine (I.Q. improved in retarded children), Phenylalanine, Tyrosine, Isoleucine.

Supplements: Evening Primrose Oil, Spirulina, Bee Pollen (contains RNA for brain), Rice Bran Syrup.

Schizophrenia

Schizophrenia is associated with nutritional deficiency, allergies, depression, tension, personality changes, fatigue and frustration. Heavy metal poisoning may be a cause of schizophrenia. It is beneficial to eliminate sugar products from the diet.

Herbal Combinations: Blood Purifier, Bone, Chelation, Nerve and Relaxation, Lower Bowels, Stress.

Single Herbs: Alfalfa, Black Cohosh, *Blue Vervain,* Capsicum, Cornsilk, Dandelion, Echinacea, Garlic, *Gotu Kola,* Hawthorn, *Hops,* Horsetail, Kelp, *Lady's Slipper, Lobelia and Mullein (together),* Mistletoe, *Papaya and Mint (together for digestion),* Parsley, Red Clover, Rose Hips, *Scullcap, Valerian,* Wood Betony, Yellow Dock.

Vitamins: A, B-complex (extra B3 and B6--essential for mental stability--B12, B15 and niacinamide), C, E.

Minerals: Multi-minerals, calcium and magnesium, iron and copper (activates brain enzymes), manganese, zinc.

Amino Acids: Free-form amino acids (keeps blood sugar level up), Glutamine, Threonine, Isoleucine (lacking in mentally ill).

Supplements: Algin, Evening Primrose Oil, Lecithin (high amounts are needed in the brain), Rice Bran Syrup, Black Currant Oil.

Senility

Slurred speech, poor memory, confusion, depression and thyroid problems can be problems dealing with senility. Toxic metal poisoning and nutritional deficiency can be causes. Many older people on drugs are labeled as senile. Liver and kidney problems are also suspected to be causes. Inner cleanse is important and exercise is vital.

Herbal Combinations: Bladder and Kidneys, Blood Purifier, Bone, Chelation, Cleansing, Digestion, General Cleanser, Glands, Immune, Liver and Gallbladder, Lower Bowels.

Single Herbs: Alfalfa, Black Cohosh, Black Walnut, Burdock, Capsicum, Chickweed, Dandelion, Echinacea, Garlic, Gentian, *Ginseng, Gotu Kola*, Hawthorn, Hops, *Ho Shou-Wu,* Irish Moss, *Kelp, Lady's Slipper,* Licorice, Lobelia, Mistletoe, Myrrh, Oregon Grape, *Pau D'Arco,* Red Clover, Rosemary, Sarsaparilla, *Scullcap,* Wood Betony, Yellow Dock, Yucca.

Vitamins: B-complex (extra B6, B12 and niacin), C, Choline, E.

Minerals: Multi-minerals, selenium, zinc.

Amino Acids: Tryptophan, Glutamine, Valine (sparks mental vigor).

Supplements: Algin, Lecithin; Goat's milk keeps you mentally alert.

Shingles

Nerve endings in the skin are affected in the shingles virus. It is a very painful disease. It is helpful to use an inner cleanse.

Herbal Combinations: Blood Purifier, Digestion, General Cleanser, Lower Bowels.

Single Herbs: *Aloe Vera,* Black Cohosh, *Black Walnut,*

Blue Vervain, Burdock, Chaparral, Chickweed, *Comfrey*, Dandelion, Echinacea, Fenugreek, Garlic, Hawthorn, *Kelp, Lady's Slipper*, Licorice, Lobelia, Oatstraw, Oregon Grape, Marshmallow, Red Clover, Rose Hips, Scullcap, White Oak, Wood Betony, Yellow Dock.

Vitamins: A, B-complex (important), C (with bioflavonoids), E.

Minerals: Calcium and magnesium (to rebuild nerves), selenium, zinc.

Amino Acids: Lysine (with vitamin C), Methionine, Cystine (detoxifies toxins).

Supplements: Aloe Vera, Liquid Chlorophyll, Rice bran syrup, Pau D'Arco lotion; Chelated cell salts, Chinese essential oils, Evening Primrose Oil or Black Currant Oil, Fish Oil Lipids, Tea Tree Oil.

Sinus Infections

Over-acid condition will cause sinus infections. Infection is involved if drainage is greenish or yellowish. Poor digestion of starch sugar and dairy products will cause runny nose. Too much of one food and eating to excess can also cause sinus infections. Allergies can cause an infection. If the drainage is clear and continues after a cold is gone, it could be allergies.

Herbal Combinations: Allergies, Blood Cleanser, Candida, Immune, Infections Lower Bowels, Lungs, Pain.

Single Herbs: Aloe Vera, Brigham Tea, Burdock, Capsicum, *Comfrey,* Echinacea, Eyebright, *Fenugreek, Garlic,* Ginger, *Golden Seal,* Hawthorn, Lobelia, Marshmallow, Mullein, *Pau D'Arco, Red Clover,* Rose Hips, *Slippery Elm, White Oak,* Yellow Dock.

Vitamins: A (lots for one month--100,000 I.U.), B-complex (extra pantothenic acid), C (with bioflavonoids).

Minerals: Multi-minerals, manganese, selenium, silicon, zinc.

Amino Acids: Lysine, Histidine, Tyrosine.

Supplements: Bee Pollen; Golden Seal snuffed up the nose; Golden Seal/Echinacea extract, chlorophyll; B-complex with vitamin C and bioflavonoids, Chelated cell salts, Evening Primrose Oil, Fish Oil Lipids, Garlic Oil, Chinese essential oils (snuffed up nose).

Skin Problems

Rashes, psoriasis and other skin problems can be caused by allergies. Many doctors are finding that a gluten-free diet helps in controlling skin rashes (wheat, barley, oats, rye). The skin is the largest elimination organ and can throw off toxins and poisons. Inner cleanse and skin brushing opens pores and eliminates dead wastes.

Herbal Combinations: Allergies, Blood Cleanser, Bone, Cleansing, Digestion, General Cleanser, Glands, Hair and Skin, Immune, Liver and Gallbladder, Lower

Bowels, Nerve and Relaxant, Potassium, Stress.

Single Herbs: *Alfalfa, Aloe Vera, Burdock,* Buchu, Capsicum, Chaparral, *Comfrey*, Cornsilk, *Dandelion,* Echinacea, Fenugreek, *Golden Seal,* Gotu Kola, Hawthorn, Hops, *Horsetail*, Ho Shou-Wu, Lady's Slipper, Lobelia, Mistletoe, *Oatstraw,* Pau D'Arco, *Queen of the Meadow*, Red Clover, Scullcap, Wood Betony, Wormwood, *Yellow Dock.*

Vitamins: A, B-complex (extra B2, B6 and niacin), D, E.

Minerals: Multi-minerals, silicon, selenium, zinc.

Amino Acids: Cysteine, Tryptophan (essential for healthy skin).

Supplements: Aloe Vera (internal and external), Evening Primrose Oil, Fish lipids, Linseed oil, Lecithin, Pau D'Arco lotion, Black Ointment (external), Chelated cell salts, Chinese Essential oils, Chlorophyll, Redmond Clay (external), Spirulina, Tea Tree Oil (externally).

Smoking

Smoking, a nicotine habit, is very addictive. It is a very serious health hazard and has been proven to cause lung cancer. It poisons the whole system. A fresh juice fast or an inner cleanse will help remove the cravings for nicotine. Tobacco is from the nightshade family which leaches calcium from the bones.

Herbal Combinations: Blood Purifier, Bone, Candida, Cleansing, Energy and Fitness, Endurance, General

Cleanse, Glands, Hypoglycemia, Immune, Lungs, Nerve and Relaxant, Lower Bowels.

Single Herbs: Alfalfa, Black Cohosh, *Chaparral,* Dandelion, Echinacea, Fenugreek, *Golden Seal, Gotu Kola,* Hawthorn, Hops, Kelp, Lady's Slipper, Licorice, Lobelia, *Passion Flower, Pau D'Arco,* Red Clover, Rose Hips, *Scullcap,* Slippery Elm, Valerian, White Willow, *Wood Betony.*

Vitamins: A (protects lungs), B-complex (builds nerves), C, E.

Minerals: Multi-minerals, selenium (protection), zinc.

Amino Acids: Free-form amino acids (keeps blood sugar level up--take between meals), Cysteine, Methionine.

Supplements: Chlorophyll, Stevia (on tongue helps cravings), Licorice extract (on tongue); B-complex with vitamin C and bioflavonoids; Black Currant Oil, Chelated cell salts, Fish oil lipids, Licorice lozenges with Zinc, Peppermint oil (on tongue to break habit), Spirulina.

Sprains

Muscle spasms, strained ligaments, tendons, swellings and cramps. Circulation needs to be increased in the injured area before healing can begin. Cold should be applied at first to prevent swelling. Fractures can be healed faster with supplements.

Herbal Combinations: Arthritis, Bone, Glands,

Immune, Nerve and Relaxant, Pain, Potassium, Stress.

Single Herbs: *Alfalfa, Aloe Vera,* Black Walnut, Capsicum, *Comfrey,* Ginger, *Golden Seal,* Hawthorn, *Hops, Horsetail,* Irish Moss, *Marshmallow, Oatstraw,* Passion Flower, Scullcap, *Slippery Elm,* Valerian, White Willow, Wood Betony, Yellow Dock.

Vitamins: A, B-complex, C (with bioflavonoids), E.

Minerals: Calcium and magnesium (more magnesium is usually needed), potassium, silicon, zinc.

Amino Acids: Lysine (helps absorption of calcium), Valine (muscle coordination), Arginine, Cystine.

Supplements: Chlorophyll, Carrot juice, Green leafy vegetables, Sesame seeds, Almonds, Black Currant Oil, Chelated cell salts (speeds healing), Chinese essential oils (externally), Fish lipids, Redmond Clay (externally).

Stress

Stress is caused by illness, injuries and life style changes--whether good or bad changes. Stress has been implicated in colitis, ulcers, strokes, cancer, high blood pressure, heart attacks, migraine headaches and nervous breakdowns. Diet and exercise are the most important to avoid stress.

Herbal Combinations: Blood Purifier, Immune, Lower Bowels, Nerves and Relaxant, Stress.

Single Herbs: *Alfalfa,* Black Cohosh, Capsicum, Catnip, *Chamomile,* Dandelion, Garlic, Ginger, Ginseng,

Golden Seal, *Gotu Kola, Hops, Kelp, Lady's Slipper*, Licorice, *Lobelia,* Mistletoe, M ullein, *Passion FLower*, Pau D'Arco, Rose Hips, Scullcap, *Valerian*, Wood Betony.

Vitamins: A, B-complex (extra B6, B12 and pantothenic acid), C (with bioflavonoids), E.

Minerals: Calcium and magnesium, potassium, iron (Yellow Dock), selenium, zinc.

Amino Acids: Cysteine, Histidine, Lysine, Tryptophan, Methionine (anti-stress), Glutamine, Arginine (increases size and activity of the thymus gland in stress).

Supplements: Evening Primrose oil, Black Currant oil, fish oil lipids, B-complex with vitamin C and bioflavonoids, chelated cell salts, Spirulina.

Teeth

Tooth decay, gum disease, and bacteria invade gums and teeth, causing infections and bone loss. To prevent infections and decay, use dental floss and brush teeth after meals (use soft toothbrush). Diet is the major cause of tooth disease.

Herbal Combinations: Bone Combination, Immune, Nerve and Relaxant, Potassium, Stress.

Single Herbs: Alfalfa, *Black Walnut, Comfrey,* Dandelion, Echinacea, Golden Seal (brush teeth with Golden Seal and Black Walnut), *Horsetail, Kelp,*

Lobelia, Marshmallow, Myrrh, Oak Bark, *Oatstraw, Pau D'Arco, Slippery Elm,* Yellow Dock.

Vitamins: A, B-complex, C (with bioflavonoids), D, E.

Minerals: Calcium and magnesium (balance), potassium, silicon, zinc.

Amino Acids: Lysine (dental caries), Aging, Histidine (essential for growth).

Supplements: Chlorophyll, Evening Primrose Oil, Black Currant Oil, Golden Seal/Echinacea extract, (rub on gums), Peppermint Oil (toothaches, Spirulina, Tea Tree oil (gum disease).

Tinnitus

Tinnitus is ringing in the ears. It can be caused from hypoglycemia, nutritional deficiencies and chemical imbalance. A hypoglycemia diet has helped many people who suffer from tinnitus.

Herbal Combinations: Blood Purifier, Hypoglycemia, Immune, Lower Bowels, Stress, Bentonite cleanse.

Single Herbs: Alfalfa, *Black Cohosh*, Black Walnut, Buchu, Burdock, Capsicum, Chaparral, Cornsilk, Dandelion, Echinacea, *Garlic*, Ginger, Ginseng, *Golden Seal, Gotu Kola, Hawthorn*, Hops, *Horsetail*, Ho Shou-Wu, Juniper Berries, Lady's Slipper, Lobelia, Parsley, Red Clover, *Scullcap, Valerian, Wood Betony*.

Vitamins: Multi-vitamin, A, B-complex, zinc.

Minerals: Multi-minerals, calcium, magnesium, selenium, silicon, zinc.

Amino Acids: Phenylalanine, Threonine, Tryptophan, Valine, Cystine, Glutamine, Histidine (hearing loss).

Supplements: Black Cohosh extract containing Chickweed, Golden Seal, Desert Tea, Licorice, Valerian and Scullcap (use in both ears); Algin, B-complex with C and bioflavonoids, Black Currant Oil, Chelated cell salts, Fish oil lipids, Garlic Oil (in ears), Peppermint oil, Lecithin (needed in head area).

Ulcers

Stress, antacids, aspirin, and many drugs can contribute to ulcers. Diet and exercise will help in stressful situations.

Herbal Combinations: Blood Purifier, Bone, Comfrey and Pepsin, Digestion, Lower Bowels, Ulcers.

Single Herbs: *Alfalfa, Aloe Vera,* Black Walnut, Burdock, *Capsicum,* Chaparral, *Comfrey,* Dandelion, Echinacea, Fenugreek, *Garlic,* Ginger, *Golden Seal,* Hawthorn, Hops, *Kelp, Lady's Slipper,* Lobelia, Myrrh, *Oatstraw, Pau D'Arco, Psyllium,* Scullcap, *Slippery Elm,* Watercress, *White Oak,* Yellow Dock.

Vitamins: A, B-complex, C (with bioflavonoids), K (alfalfa), E, U (cabbage juice).

Minerals: Calcium and magnesium balance, selenium, silicon, zinc.

Amino Acids: Histidine, Lysine, Tryptophan, Glutamine, (heals peptic ulcer).

Supplements: Aloe Vera Juice, Liquid Chlorophyll, Glucomannan, Evening Primrose Oil, Black Currant Oil, Fish Oil Lipids, Chelated Cell Salts, Garlic Oil.

Varicose Veins

Pregnancy, constipation, lack of exercise, obesity, or poor diet can contribute to varicose veins. Hemorrhoids are enlarged veins around the anus. When blood vessels are weak in the rectal area and allowed to become worse it can cause prolapses of the anal wall, rupturing the veins and causing infections. Avoid constipation at all times.

Herbal Combinations: Blood Purifier, Bone, Chelation, Colitis, Digestion, Glands, Liver and Gallbladder, Lower Bowels, Bentonite Cleanse.

Single Herbs: Alfalfa, Aloe Vera, Bayberry, Black Walnut Buckthorn, *Butcher's Broom, Capsicum,* Cascara Sagrada (colon rebuilder), Chaparral, Comfrey, *Golden Seal, Horsetail, Kelp (strengthens veins),* Lobelia, Mullein Oil (relieves pain), *Oatstraw, Parsley,* Pau D'Arco, Red Raspberry, Slippery Elm, Uva Ursi, *White Oak Bark (strengthens veins), Witch Hazel,* Wood Betony.

Vitamins: B-complex (extra B6 and B12), C (with

bioflavonoids), D, K (alfalfa), E.

Minerals: Multi-minerals, calcium and magnesium (balance), manganese, selenium, silicon, zinc.

Amino Acids: Lysine (strengthens circulation), Methionine (eliminates toxins), Phenylalanine (blood vessels), Arginine (cleans veins), Cystine (detoxifies), Histidine (cleanses).

Supplements: Bee Pollen, Glucomannan, Lecithin, Liquid Chlorophyll, Oak Bark Poultice, Psyllium, Chelated Cell Salts, Fish Oil Lipids, Nutritional Fiber Supplement, Redmond Clay (external), Spirulina.

Venereal Disease

Venereal disease is a contagious sexually transmitted disease. Syphilis and gonorrhea are the most common types of venereal diseases.

Herbal Combinations: Blood Purifier, Candida, Cleansing, General Cleanser, Immune, Infections, Lower Bowels, Parasites and Worms, Stress, Bentonite Cleanse.

Single Herbs: Alfalfa, Aloe Vera, *Black Walnut,* Buchu, *Burdock*, Capsicum, Chaparral, Comfrey, *Echinacea,* Eyebright, Fenugreek, *Garlic, Gentian, Golden Seal,* Hawthorn, Horsetail, *Kelp,* Licorice, Lobelia, Marshmallow, *Oatstraw,* Parsley, *Pau D'Arco,* Queen of the Meadow, *Red Clover*, Red Raspberry, Slippery Elm, Squaw Vine, Uva Ursi, White Oak, Yarrow, Yellow Dock.

Vitamins: A, C (with bioflavonoids), K, E.

Minerals: Multi-minerals, selenium, zinc.

Amino Acids: Free-form amino acids (all are needed), extra sulphur amino acids: Cysteine, Taurine, Tryptophan, Glycine, Glutamic Acid, Lysine.

Supplements: Acidophilus, Chlorophyll, Black Walnut Extract (internally and externally); Black Currant Oil, Chelated Cell Salts, Fish Oil Lipids, Garlic Oil, Golden Seal/Echinacea Extract (external and internal), Spirulina, Tea Tree Oil (external).

Warts

Warts are considered a viral infection.

Herbal Combinations: Blood Purifier, Bone, Cleansing, General Cleanser, Glands, Immune, Lower Bowels.

Single Herbs: *Aloe Vera,* Bayberry, Burdock, *Black Walnut*, Chickweed, Comfrey, Dandelion, Echinacea, Fenugreek, *Garlic, Golden Seal,* Lobelia, Oatstraw, Oregon Grape, Pau D'Arco, Red Clover, White Oak, Yellow Dock.

Vitamins: A, B-complex, C (with bioflavonoids), E used internally and externally).

Minerals: Multi-minerals, potassium, selenium, silicon, zinc.

Amino Acids: Cysteine, Taurine, Tryptophan, Glutamic Acid, Lysine.

Supplements: Chlorophyll, Wheatgrass Juice, Black Walnut Extract (externally), Tea Tree Oil (applied externally), Chinese Oils (external); make a paste with apple cider vinegar and capsicum, put on wart and cover with bandaid™.

Wounds

Wounds, abrasions, cuts, bruises.

Herbal Combinations: Blood Purifier, Bone Combination (external and internal), Cleansing, Immune, Infection.

Single Herbs: *Aloe Vera, Black Walnut,* Burdock, Capsicum, Chickweed, *Comfrey,* Echinacea, *Fenugreek (poultice),* Garlic, *Golden Seal,* Horsetail, Lobelia. *Marshmallow (poultice),* Myrrh, *Plantain,* Red Clover, Sarsaparilla, *Slippery Elm,* St. Johnswort, *White Oak,* White Willow, *Witch Hazel,* Wood Betony, Yarrow.

Vitamins: A, B-complex, C, E.

Minerals: Calcium, selenium, zinc.

Amino Acids: Cystine (assists wound healing), Proline (heals wounds).

Supplements: For bruises use Black Walnut, Comfrey and Aloe Vera Juice (apply externally); for infections use

Aloe Vera, Slippery Elm, and White Willow; to stop bleeding use Cayenne extract or powder; to prevent infections and to stop pain use salves containing Comfrey.

2

CLEANSING AND IMMUNE DIETS

Cleansing Diets

Cleansing diets are very beneficial to the health and well-being of the body. They are very effective during colds, flu or illness. They will help clean and purify the body of excess mucus and toxins. The body has the ability to rid itself of toxins if it is given the chance. Toxins are expelled through the skin (which needs to be kept clean and scrubbed), nose, mouth, stomach and colon. The purpose of cleansing is to eliminate excessive mucus and toxins. Under normal circumstances, mucus is a normal secretion of the body's mucous membranes to keep the lining of throat, nose and alimentary canal lubricated. Excess mucus is thick, sticky and cloudy and attracts toxins, viruses, germs, and worms and parasites. The wrong kind of mucus is produced in the digestive tract, lymphatic system, bowels, lungs, reproductive organs and connective tissues.

A toxic body creates an atmosphere where germs accumulate and viruses can live and cause all kinds of diseases. A toxic body causes allergies, cancer, arthritis, cysts, depression and many other diseases that we are faced with today.

One must be prepared mentally before undertaking

any new cleansing fast or change of diet. One has to want to feel better, or get well badly enough to want to change their present diet. Many people can testify of the benefits of changing their eating habits and going on a cleansing fast. They feel better physically and mentally.

A cleansing diet will produce unpleasant side effects. When undertaking a cleansing diet, your body will crave all the junk foods you have ever eaten. You will have strong urges to eat sweet foods, or whatever food you have eaten in the past. It could produce headaches, fatigue, nausea, depression, gas, bloating, or many other symptoms.

One very common side effect when cleansing the body is a general overall bad feeling. If you prepare yourself mentally, then you will be better equipped to cope with it if it happens. If you are not prepared for the unpleasant side effects you will want to toss in the towel and give up all together because you can convince yourself that this diet is making you sick.

When the body is cleansing it dumps toxins into the bloodstream and produces unpleasant feelings until all the toxins are eliminated. It will be well worth all you have to endure during a cleansing diet. You will feel so good you will want to kick your heels up and dance. You will also want to kick yourself for not doing a cleanse sooner.

Cleansing Diet:
Herbs and Lemon Water Diet

Between meals drink the grain drink (coffee substitute), Red Clover Blend, Pau D'Arco, Apple Cinnamon Tea, Buchu Tea or Red Raspberry Tea.

This is a cleansing diet while still eating. This is a diet for beginners and those who have to work. You can eat while on this cleanse if you eat only the foods listed. You can do this up to three months. Then you need to rest your body and use the immune diet. This is a wonderful cleanse (my very favorite), and has been very effective for me and others who have used it.

Breakfast

One half hour before breakfast: One teaspoon of psyllium hulls in a glass of pure lemon water using one tablespoon of fresh lemon juice. Take two parasite combinations, two comfrey and pepsin, two blood cleanser, and two lower bowel cleansers. Some people need to add one or two cascara sagrada before going to bed at night. Use your own good judgement on what your body needs. If cramping or nausea is a problem add two ginger capsules. Adjust this to fit your needs. There are people who take four of each herb an get excellent results. But always take it slow to begin with.

If cleansing seems to be too fast for you, then slow down. Take less of the herbs and eat more food. This cleanse is designed to clean slowly. It is also designed to adjust to the individual because everyone is different. Remember if you eat meat on this cleanse you will stop the cleanse and the good it is doing. Meat has a tendency to plug up the system as it throws uric acid back into the blood stream

For breakfast eat fruit only, up to one half a pound of: apples, apricots, grapes, cherries, papayas, peaches, pears, pineapples, plums, persimmons, berries and melons of all kinds, but eat them alone; reconstituted dried fruit such as dates, figs, prunes or raisin; unsulfured.

Lunch

One half hour before lunch use lemon juice, psyllium and herbs.

Lunch should be the largest meal of the day. Use one cup brown rice and millet cooked together, or one cup millet and buckwheat, or one cup brown rice with buckwheat. Season with vegetable seasoning, kelp and a little raw butter. Chew this very well because the enzymes to digest the grains are in the mouth; if you do not chew well you may have indigestion. Also make a vegetable salad with any five of the following vegetables (raw vegetable only): Leaf lettuce, asparagus, green beans, beets, broccoli, brussel sprouts, carrots, cauliflower, cucumbers, celery, endive, fresh corn, onions, parsley, Jerusalem artichokes, parsnips, radishes, rutabagas, spinach, sprouts (all kinds), squash, swiss chard, tomatoes and turnips. Use fresh lemon and olive oil to season.

If you are still hungry add some lightly steamed vegetables--artichokes, carrots, potatoes (red), broccoli, cauliflower or winter squash.

Supper

One half hour before supper use lemon juice, psyllium and herbs.

Eat raw vegetable soups *(Today's Healthy Eating,* page 166) and a raw salad, or baked potato with mock sour cream and a raw salad, or one cup brown rice, millet or buckwheat and a raw salad.

Before going to bed take the outlined herbs in plain water. Also you may want to take some herbs for the nervous system: Nerve combinations, hops, passion flower, scullcap or lady's slipper.

Immune Diet

An immune diet is a balanced diet that will fortify the immune system and protect the body from disease as well as provide nutrients for energy. A balanced diet will balance body weight, and keep it under control. A balanced diet will fill protein needs. Protein is essential for health. If you eat enough natural foods to satisfy your hunger, you will usually get enough protein required for the body. Protein is in all natural foods and it is felt that the amino acids (derived from protein) can be stored and released by the body as needed. One meal high in certain amino acids can compensate for a meal eaten days or weeks earlier which was deficient in that missing amino acid.

Balanced Diet

Grains: Buckwheat, millet, brown rice, wheat, triticale, cornmeal, oats, rye and barley.

Legume's: Beans and peas; black-eyed peas, split green and yellow peas, beans (garbanzo, pinto, white, kidney, auki, soy, black, red and mung). Add lentils and tofu. Beans can be sprouted before cooking.

Vegetables: Eat vegetables of all colors--yellow, orange, dark green, red and white; sprouts of all kinds, artichoke, beets, beet greens, bell peppers, brussel sprouts, cabbage, carrots, cauliflower, celery, chinese cabbage, collard greens, corn, cucumbers, eggplant, Jerusalem artichokes, leeks, leaf lettuce, mushrooms, okra, onions, parsley, parsnips, peas, potatoes, radishes, spinach, string beans, summer squash, sweet potatoes, tomatoes, turnips, winter squash, yams and zucchini; I also enjoy spaghetti squash with butter and grated parmesan cheese, or with a tomato sauce; if you use the nightshade family (potatoes, tomatoes, eggplant and peppers) the diet should include dairy products (such as cheese, sour cream, etc.).

Fruits: Whole fruits, eaten according to season when possible, such as apples, apricots, avocados, bananas, berries, cherries, citrus fruit (tree ripened is best), coconuts, dates, figs, grapes, papaya, and all fruit.

Dairy Products: Butter, raw cow's milk, raw goats milk, sour cream and raw cheese occasionally.

Nuts and Seeds: Raw nuts--almonds, brazil nuts, cashews, hazelnuts, pecans, pine nuts, pistachio, pumpkin, sesame and sunflower seeds and walnuts; flax seeds and chia seeds are also very nutritious.

Fats and Oils: Unsaturated fats, cold-pressed oils, safflower, sesame, sunflower and olive oil; use often evening primrose oil, black currant oil, and fish oil lipids.

Animal Protein: They can be eaten occasionally for an immune diet: eggs, chicken, turkey (without skin) and fish.

3

COLON HEALTH

The type of diet you eat will determine the nature of the bacteria in the intestine. The colon cannot be efficient in its proper function if the diet has consisted mostly of processed food (fried or overcooked), white sugar, white flour products and white rice which takes longer to travel through the colon than fibrous foods, and gives any cancer agent longer to act on the bowel wall. A diet high in animal protein promotes bacterial growth which changes harmless amino acids and transforms them into very strong and powerful toxins. Many of these toxins pass through the liver almost entirely unchanged and either enter the bloodstream to find a weakened spot in the body to do its job. Fatigue, nervous irritability, intestinal disorders, headaches and many other problems develop.

When these processed foods coat the inner walls of the colon they become encrusted. This accumulation of stagnant material coating the walls of the colon needs to be softened and loosened so it can be eliminated from the system. This material cannot be eliminated if the same diet is continued.

Autointoxication is the process whereby the body poisons itself by harboring a cesspool of decaying matter in its colon. It contains a high concentration of harmful bacteria. The toxins released by the decay process get into the bloodstream and go to all parts of the body and weaken the entire system. The weakest part of the body will suffer.

Before World War II it was typical for physicians to make statements about autointoxication as being the most important primary and contributing causes of many disorders and diseases of the human body. Many articles were written in medical journals about intestinal toxemia and autointoxication. This idea has been abandoned by the medical profession in favor of drugs and surgery. The typical American diet has deteriorated so badly that it breeds bacteria and causes intestinal toxemia.

A normal healthy colon has the function of proper absorption, assimilation and utilization of nutrients from the foods we eat as well as the elimination of waste material. Colon cleanse will have a lasting effect on any ailment, sickness, or disease.

Colonics and Enemas

Colonics are colon irrigations administered by a trained operator who uses many gallons of water in a very controlled atmosphere. It is very important that the person is a knowledgeable, trained operator and is with you during the whole procedure, which takes approximately thirty minutes. It is considered a very thorough and sophisticated enema.

If a person feels rotten and has built-up toxins as well as problems of the colon, then periodic colonics are an essential way to clean out the entire colon and bring it to its proper function again.

Colon cleansing works faster if you take herbs orally to loosen up the built-up material on the colon walls. The use of enemas or colonics will help to remove old built-up toxins as soon as they are loosened. Just using herbs orally causes the material to be dissolved, but can cause constipation if it isn't removed when it is loosened. It is very important to remember to remove all loosened material from the colon as quickly as possible, whether using herbs, liquids, enemas or colonics.

The reluctance to accept enemas is brought about by ignorance of their function and purpose. The enema helps to relieve stress, provides a clean colon, and gives a sense of well being. The enema helps with the proper removal of toxins and debris from the colon, so nutrients can be absorbed properly and to help keep diseases from taking hold of the body. Almost any ailment can be helped with cleansing the colon.

How To Take An Enema

Use a regular enema bag or a hospital disposable bag. The bag should not be over 18 inches higher than the body as the enema solution would run into the colon too fast and cause discomfort. Lubricate the tube with vitamin E or lubricant jelly.

The knee-chest position is very efficient and many people prefer this method. Their head, shoulders and arms are on the floor with the buttocks elevated. Another position is lying on the left side, letting in about one cup of enema solution at a time. Massage gently on the left side of the abdomen, working down in the direction of the rectum. Massage the right side. Turn over on the back for about five minutes, then on the right side. Try to retain the enema for about 15 minutes or longer if you can, then it can be expelled. Remove the colon tube, stay on the left side for a few minutes.

Control the enema tube and allow as much as is comfortable. When to expel is determined by cramping and also the urgency to expel. The ability to hold more will come as the colon is cleansed. Only use purified water.

Types of Enemas

Garlic Enema: Six garlic bulbs in the cups of pure water, blend, strain. Use 1/2 cup of this mixture in 2 quarts of water. Garlic is nature's antibiotic. It helps relieve stress and kills parasites, while cleansing toxins from the colon.

Catnip Enema: Steep two tablespoons catnip in a quart of pure water, strain and add to enema bag with more pure water. Catnip is soothing to the colon, helps children in colic, fevers, and childhood diseases.

Slippery Elm: Use one quart of pure water in blender with two tablespoons slippery elm powder, strain, add to enema bag with more water. Neutralizes acidity and absorbs foul gases. Acts as a buffer against irritations in the colon. Good for colitis, diarrhea and hemorrhoids.

Flaxseed Tea: Boil 1/4 cup flaxseeds in one quart of pure water. Strain and add more water to the enema bag.

Special Dietary Helps

Vitamin A: Important in maintaining strong healthy cells. Needs a steady supply to strengthen and repair the tissues. Needed to support mucous membrane linings.

Acidophilus: Taken orally is beneficial in detoxifying the bowel as well as building the friendly bacteria. Very beneficial for healthy bowels.

Agar Agar: Is widely used as a thickener and emulsifier. It is very beneficial for constipation. It swells to many times its bulk when it reaches the intestines and helps increase the peristaltic action without causing painful griping. Mixes with the food intake and moves it out.

Alfalfa: Very nourishing and provides the bowels with bulk material which gets into the pockets of the bowels to keep them clean.

Aloe Vera: Very good for colon health; use with ginger to prevent griping.

Apples: With their fruit-acid salts, apples stimulate the digestive processes--good for constipation. The cellulose content helps soften the partly digested food in the intestines.

Bentonite (Hydrated): Absorbs and neutralizes toxins and bacteria found in the alimentary canal and detoxifies it.

Black Walnut: Kills parasites in the colon and other areas of the body.

Bran: Unprocessed bran increases stool weight and reduces the transit time of food. It stabilizes intestinal regularity without irritating. Removes waste from the bowels. Always use with a large glass of water. Nourishes the colon.

Brewers Yeast: Rich in the amino acids and all the B-complex vitamins.

Buckwheat: Provides bulk in the colon. Sprouted is the best.

Buttermilk: Contains lactic acid for bowel tone. Soothing to the nervous system and the bowels.

Vitamin C: Very important to control the sievability of the cells. Needed for healthy mucous membranes.

Calcium: Aids the body's utilization of iron, regulates the passage of nutrients in and out of the cell wall. The most abundant mineral in the body. Good for the nerves.

Chlorophyll: Healing and cleansing for the colon. It helps stop growth of toxic bacteria in the bowels, and encourages normal growth of friendly bacteria.

Comfrey: Healing and soothing to the bowels.

Enzymes: Taken at bedtime will help complete digestion of food left in the colon.

Exercise: Lack of exercise can cause a lazy colon. Exercise strengthens the colon, produces natural lactic acid when you exercise.

Figs: Figs, prunes and raisins are all good for bowel health. Soak overnight in juice or pure water for best results. Figs are good especially when eaten fresh. High in natural sugar, the seeds have a laxative coating.

Flaxseed: Used internally, helps furnish bulk to the bowels. Used as tea for enemas, relives inflammation in the bowels, as well as cleaning out toxins.

Ginger: Wonderful herb for nausea and stomach cramps and to prevent spasms and flatulence. Contains elements to destroy parasites in the colon.

Hydrochloric Acid: Helps in protein assimilation as well as fasts and carbohydrates.

Iron: A deficiency in iron may be related to toxins and poor elimination. Avoid inorganic iron, as it oxidizes vitamin E and makes it ineffective.

Laxatives: Interfere with the proper absorption of important sodium and potassium balance in the large intestine. Potassium is lost when laxatives are taken.

Lemon & Water: Taken first thing in the morning helps clean bowels and stomach.

Licorice: Helps reduce flatulence and is soothing to the lining of the stomach and intestinal tract.

Lymphatic System: The colon is the principal organ for the detoxification of the lymph glands. Rebound exercise helps remove toxins from the lymph glands. Echinacea, red clover and mullein are herbs that clean the lymphatics.

Meat: Avoid meat for a healthy colon--contains very strong purifying materials. It spoils in the intestinal tract faster than any other food.

Magnesium: Necessary in the digestion of food, tones muscles, helps in depression.

Millet: High in protein, provides fiber for the colon, easily assimilated.

Pantothenic Acid: Up to 50 mg. daily has helped restore function in paralysis of the colon.

Papaya: Use after eating--especially if you eat meat. It will digest meat better than anything else.

Potassium: diarrhea as well as stress can cause loss. Needed to help balance body fluids.

Sesame Seeds: Easily assimilated. Fiber for the colon.

Psyllium Hulls: Provides bulk and lubrication to the bowels. It expands when taken with water to create bulk and remove intestinal putrefaction.

Sprouting: Seeds and grains sprouted increase the nutrients hundreds of times.

Stress: Can cause colon tightening, poor digestion and assimilation. Prolonged stress can cause constipation, lead to diarrhea and diverticulitis.

Toxins: The brain suffers. Toxins interfere with chemical balance of the body.

Yogurt: Provides friendly bacteria in the bowels, helps build immunity to disease.

Zinc: Large amounts have proven to be healing to the colon. Healing to chronic ulceration of epithelial tissues. 15-30 mg. daily, even more at times.

Fiber Foods

Alfalfa seeds	Carob	Millet-oats, steel cut
Almonds	Chia Seeds	Pinto beans
Barley	Corn-grains	Rye
Blackeyed peas	Flaxseeds	Soybeans
Bran	Garbanzo Beans	Split peas
Brown rice	Lentils	Sunflower Seeds
Buckwheat	Mung Beans	Whole Wheat

Seed Cereal For Colon

1 T. ground sesame seeds
1 T. ground sunflower seeds
1 T. ground almonds
1 tsp chia seeds
1 tsp flaxseeds

Add two tablespoons of currants, raisins, or chopped dried apricots. Add raw apple juice or pineapple juice to cover. Set overnight in refrigerator. Ready to eat in the morning. (Excerpts from *Today's Healthy Eating*, by Louise Tenney).

4

INFERTILITY

A Growing Concern

Infertility is becoming a problem for those who desire to have children. Over two million couples want to have children and find that they are unable to conceive. There are many doctors specializing in infertility. The cost of tests for the wife as well as the husband is expensive and time consuming with no guarantee of success.

There are many reasons for infertility. The female may have tubes that are blocked, ovulation problems, hormonal imbalance, or weak uterus. The male can have low sperm count, immature sperm incapable of fertilization and many more problems that account for the inability to conceive. It is well known that malnutrition can cause sterility. Good nutrition is essential in the male and female for fertility. We know that during times of famine women have a far less chance of conceiving. It is as if the natural order of life prevents conceiving when the environment of the baby could be harmed. Many of our youth who have Anorexia Nervosa have ceased their menstrual flow. Women who join the service and have increased strenuous exercise have ceased menstruating-- especially during the first year of training.

We are now seeing many doctors who are very concerned about how important nutrition is during pregnancy in the development of a healthy baby. More than ever before it has been shown that improving the health of the female increases her vitality and improves the quality of the offspring. A large amount of money is spent on research devoted to pregnancy and nutrition. But now much time and money is spent on research of infertility and nutrition? Wouldn't it be wise to look into the possibility of nutrition playing a major role in infertility before a lot of time and money is spent on tests, surgery, fertility pills and many other drugs? The declining birth rate in Europe in the past fifty years was linked to the removal of vitamins B and E from grains during the milling process. If we looked seriously at the eating habits of those who are infertile in the United States today we would see a link between diet and the inability to conceive. I am not saying that it would solve all the problems that couples have in conceiving but it would do a great deal of good for the general health of the couple trying to have a family.

Special Dietary Helps

Vitamin A: Vitamin A is essential for maintaining healthy epithelial tissues. The uterus is lined with epithelial tissues and when there is a deficiency there can be degeneration or keratinization (roughening and hardening) of the placenta. Vitamin A is indispensable in pregnancy and lactation. It assists in maintaining normal glandular activity. Sterility is one of the deficiency symptoms of vitamin A.

B-Complex Vitamins: B-complex vitamins are vital for both mental and physical health. B1 (Thiamine) is indispensible for pregnancy and lactation. Lack of this vitamin can cause defective reproductive function. B2 (Riboflavin) deficiency can cause retarded and defective growth and brain disorders. B5 (niacin) aids in energy metabolism and the utilization of fats and protein. Effective against toxemia of pregnancy. B6 plays an important role in the utilization of zinc, and other minerals. Protects against stress; helps in nausea, edema, toxemia. Stabilizes female hormone levels which is critical in conceiving. B9 (Folic Acid), is necessary for the division of all body cells and for the production of the substances which carry out hereditary patterns, RNA and DNA. Without it, no growth can take place. B12 (Riboflavin) helps to stimulate B9, B6, B12 and plays an important role in energy release.

Birth Control Pills: The Pill was developed about 30 years ago. Most women have taken the Pill without fear, and were convinced that it was safe and harmless.

Women took to The Pill as eagerly as they took to the Thalidomide Drug with confidence that since it was prescribed by their doctors it was safe and free from side effects. The Pill manufacturers are faced with hundreds of lawsuits from women who were convinced the Pill was safe. Oral contraceptives are unsafe drugs with numerous side effects. The Pill can cause permanent infertility, high blood pressure, blood clots, strokes, heart disease, kidney failure, varicose veins, and cancer of the breast, uterus and liver. These are just a few of the dangerous side effects of the Pill. The B vitamins are also depleted by continuous use of the Pill. Iron and Zinc are two of the most vital minerals to help counteract the damaging effects of the Pill. Adding kelp to the diet will counteract any damage the Pill has done.

Selenium and Iodine also should be added to help counteract the Pill's side effects. Iodine is found abundantly in kelp.

Vitamin C: Vitamin C is an essential vitamin to take every day along with bioflavonoids to help protect the body from germs and viruses. Lack of vitamin C can cause varicose veins, slow healing of wounds, frequent colds and other illnesses.

Calcium: Most women are deficient in calcium, about 1500 mg. is needed daily. It is necessary for growth, repairs and maintenance of nerves, bones and teeth. It calms nerves, builds blood and promotes growth. A lack can cause menstrual disorders and restlessness. A stronger dosage is required during pregnancy so it is logical more calcium is needed to become pregnant.

Vitamin D: Vitamin D is essential in pregnancy to prevent rickets in infants. If there is a severe deficiency in the mother, nature would likely prevent conception. It is essential to regulate absorption and metabolism of bone forming elements, calcium and phosphorus. Lack can cause restlessness, irritability and insomnia.

Vitamin E: Vitamin E is called the fertility vitamin for the male as well as the female. The prostate gland contains a high concentration of vitamin E. The pituitary gland also contains high amounts of vitamin E which helps to regulate ovulation. Lack of vitamin E is the major cause of premature babies. Vitamin E helps to prevent miscarriage, and increases male and female fertility.

Chromium: Low chromium levels can be associated with low production and fertility. Chromium works well with the B-complex vitamins. It is not common to find a chromium deficiency, but if there are other deficiencies it could make a difference.

Drugs: Prescription drugs, over-the-counter and street drugs. They can be very dangerous to the reproductive organs.

Foods To Eat: Change to a wholesome diet. More fresh fruit and vegetables. Use more grains and vegetable salads. Use raw nuts, seeds. Cook more beans, peas, lentils. Use millet and buckwheat often. They are alkaline foods to help restore balance from too much acid foods. Use sprouts often in salads, alfalfa, mung beans, fenugreek and more.

Glands: Mini-trampoline exercises will help clean and stimulate the lymphatic glands. Properly nourished glands will keep the hormone secretion regular. The Hypothalamus is the organ in the brain that produces the hormone necessary for regulating the normal menstrual cycle. The Pituitary Gland is located at the base of the skull and controls the female hormones estrogen and progesterone which are secreted by the ovaries. Herbs to nourish the glands are: Echinacea, Sarsaparilla, Lobelia, Black Walnut, Chaparral, Golden Seal, Red Clover, Licorice, and Yellow Dock.

Herbs For Fertility: Red Raspberry strengthens the uterus. It contains iron and calcium, and other minerals to help build the blood. It aids digestion. It is beneficial for prolapsed uterus and leucorrhea. Good for hemorrhoids. Alfalfa is very rich in minerals, as well as vitamins. Oatstraw is good for any uterine problems. Red Clover helps to balance estrogen; helps in any vaginal infection. False Unicorn has been used in infertility and impotence. It helps to create a healthful pure environment in the body. An excellent herb to put the body in a healthy state to promote conception. Licorice has helped to increase fertility around ovulation. Sarsaparilla stimulates progesterone action, the lack of which can inhibit ovulation.

Hypothyroidism: The thyroid gland is closely linked with reproduction. It is known that the gland becomes enlarged in women at puberty and with pregnancy. Thyroid secretions appear to be essential for the development of the egg and for proper ovarian secretions. If thyroid function is low an egg may be discharged from an ovary but it may not be fertilizable or if fertilized, may not be capable of nesting so that pregnancy is quickly aborted. (Dr. Broda O. Barnes, M.D., *Hypothyroidism: The Unsuspected Illness*, Page 129).

Iodine: Essential for reproduction. Found in natural kelp or dulse. It has been found that women with a low thyroid cannot conceive. Lack of iodine can cause retardation in a fetus. Disturbed iodine metabolism often causes sterility.

Iron: It is an essential nutrient; the need is increased considerably during pregnancy, so may be necessary in getting pregnant. Yellow dock and dandelion together build blood. Liquid chlorophyll and vitamin C tend to increase iron absorption.

Manganese: Along with zinc will help activate enzyme action. It helps to maintain normal reproductive process. Deficiency can cause sterility as well as defective reproduction function.

Meat: Animal food tends to have more pesticides than plant food. Poisons are retained longer in animal fat than in plant tissues. The Environmental Protection Agency found chemical residue in plant foods as well as in animal food. The amounts, on the average, were one-tenth of those found in flesh foods. Meat is hard to digest and will accumulate in the body as uric acid and toxic waste material.

Minerals: A good mineral supplement has a positive effect in fertility. Especially iodine, manganese, copper and zinc. The link between trace elements and normal reproduction is very strong.

Pantothenic Acid (part of the B vitamins): Lack of has shown to cause the male to become sterile, and females to give birth to deformed babies or to miscarry.

Protein: A very essential nutrient for life and growth. The amino acids of which protein is made from found in plant food is the same structure whether it comes from beans or T-bone steak. Protein can be obtained from grains, legume's, seeds, nuts, sprouts, cheese, and eggs. Powdered protein supplements help to supply more needed protein to the body.

Selenium: This mineral works with vitamin E, and has now been found essential for health. Protects against harmful oxidation and free radical formation. Protects against cancer cells.

Slant Board: The slant board is the only way to exercise the uterus. Gravity is constantly pulling the uterus and a slant board would help pull and eliminate strain on the uterus.

Smoking: Smoking increases the risk of stillbirth, miscarriage late in pregnancy, and deaths of babies right after birth. Toxic material and inhaled smoke are transmitted through the placenta to the unborn baby. Smoking decreases the blood flow to the fetus. Carbon monoxide found in cigarette smoke decreases oxygen flow to the mother and into the placenta where the baby is fed. Cigarette smoke also contains chemicals that cause cancer. These chemicals enter the fetal bloodstream when the mother smokes during pregnancy and can cause cancer in the unborn baby, which may manifest itself later in the child.

Stress: Stress and anxiety can upset regular menstrual cycle. Stress depletes nutrients from the body. It is usually the nutrients that are necessary to get pregnant such as vitamin A, C, B vitamins and E. Stress will cause the weakest part of the body to be affected. Stress can cause female problems and therefore cause infertility.

Zinc: A necessary mineral for the sex organs. It is important in the sperm count in the male. Zinc is found in high concentration in the prostate.

5

PREGNANCY

It is essential to gain knowledge of the importance of nutrients in the body before you decide to get pregnant. Whatever you take into the body has an effect on the fetus. The food you eat is what creates the substance of the baby. Too much sugar puts stress on the pancreas of the mother as well as on the pancreas of the baby. (Excess sugar robs the body of the mother as well as the baby of vitamins and minerals essential for the development of the baby, especially the B vitamins. Excess sugar can cause hypoglycemia in the baby).

Pregnancy can be a very happy experience if the mother's body is free from toxins. Toxins can cause nausea and hormonal imbalances. Cleansing the colon and the liver will help to avoid any undue nausea during pregnancy.

Special Dietary Helps

Vitamin A: Builds resistance to disease, promotes growth, protects against toxins. Aids in the growth of strong bones, along with calcium and vitamin C.

Alcohol: Avoid during pregnancy. Alcohol passes freely through the placenta. It becomes toxic when used in quantities in excess of the organisms ability to metabolize it. It can cause fetal alcohol syndrome and small stature, small head, narrow eye slits, flattened nasal bridge, receding chin, mental retardation and cardial defects. Drinking can affect the baby even before conception.

Alfalfa: Very rich in calcium and magnesium balance. Excellent food for mother-to-be as well as nursing to promote rich milk for the baby. High in vitamin K which clots the blood and prevents hemorrhages. Contains enzymes to help assimilation and digestion of food.

Almonds: Raw almonds are an excellent source of protein. Helps promote normal bowel function. Almond milk is good for inflamed stomach and intestines. It is rich in calcium. To make almond milk, soak one cup of almonds overnight. Then put the almonds in a blender with 4 cups of pure water and blend until it looks like milk--about three minutes. Add a little honey or pure maple syrup. Use on cereals, granola and in sauces instead of milk.

Anemia: It is very common during pregnancy. If there are problems with the assimilation and digestion the iron may not be utilized. Digestion will be helped if papaya, alfalfa, and enzyme tablets are taken along with the iron herbs, Dandelion and Yellow Dock.

B-Complex Vitamins: Essential to build up the immune system. Helps to avoid infections of the vagina. The B vitamins help protect the body from exhaustion and irritability. Extra B6 helps keep down swelling and prevents nausea. 300 mg. in the morning and 300 mg. at night have been helpful for some people. Extra B12 provides more energy. Builds the body against allergies, strengthens the brain and heart, and helps in enzymatic function.

Brown Rice: Provides the B vitamins--provides energy.

Beans: Pinto helps to leach out toxic metals (sprout before cooking).

Vitamin C Complex: C (with bioflavonoids) and zinc helps to enhance contractions and minimize stretch marks. It helps to keep viruses under control during pregnancy. It will protect the growing embryo from virus particles in the mother's tissues. Massive doses of C have been successful in treating acute attacks of viral diseases. 1,000 to 15,000 daily, with bioflavonoids, will help prevent bacterial infections, and help the liver to detoxify the system.

Calcium: Pregnant women require more calcium. Deficiency is caused by high-protein diet, especially meat. Calcium protects against toxic environment. Calcium and iron are very deficient minerals in women's diets, so it is essential to add natural supplements during pregnancy. Calcium provides proper development of the bones in the fetus.

Chemicals: Avoid especially during pregnancy-- preservatives, additives, food coloring, pesticides, and any unnatural substances like MSG; read labels. Wash fruits and vegetables before eating. Chemicals overwork the liver, which is already stressed because of pregnancy.

Chlorophyll: Obtained through green drinks, sprouts, wheat grass juice or liquid chlorophyll. Very beneficial during pregnancy. Builds blood. Anaerobic bacteria, a disease-producing micro-organism living within many human bodies, cannot live in the presence of oxygen or oxygen-producing agents such as chlorophyll. It is considered a protection to the body. Chlorophyll possesses the properties to break down poisonous carbon dioxide as well as released free oxygen. Chlorophyll was discovered to be similar to that of hemoglobin (red cells) in human blood.

Constipation: Common during pregnancy because the same hormone that maintains your pregnancy also makes your intestines less active. In order to increase absorption of nutrients for the growing baby: Drink pure water. Eat fiber food: Bran, whole grain, nuts and seeds (sunflower, sesame, chia, flax), barley, brown rice, buckwheat, corn, millet, oats, and rye.

Vitamin D: Essential to help calcium to absorb. Very vital to bone and tooth development. Helps development of jaw bones so that the teeth have room for proper growth.

Drugs: Should be avoided at all times, but especially during the first three months of pregnancy. Aspirin interferes with the clotting of blood, so bleeding could develop. It also interferes with uterine contractions and could delay labor. Antibiotics interfere with the production of RNA and protein, and could cause damage to the fetus. Drugs can cause problems in the newborn baby, such as jaundice, respiratory problems, deformed limbs, mental retardation, loss of appetite. DES given to pregnant women to prevent miscarriages showed up in the child after they were grown. The daughters are showing high risks of miscarriages, tubal pregnancy, stillbirth and premature births. Caffeine passes the placental barrier and into the baby's blood, interfering with the growth and development. It can also interfere with DNA repair, delays labor and inhibits uterine contractions. Heavy drugs such as heroin and cocaine when taken during pregnancy expose their unborn babies to serious harm. The infants can be born addicted, which is a very pitiful sight.

Fluids: Herb teas (red raspberry) and pure water help the liver to detoxify, and help prevent constipation.

Fruit: Eat lots of fresh fruit during pregnancy. Apples are a cleanser of the body, for they help to eliminate toxins. Bananas are high in potassium, but use very ripe. Best to use the fruit when it is in season. Organically grown if possible.

Exercise: Helps for easier delivery. Helps the lymph glands to clean the system.

Vitamin E: 800 units a day have been recommended by nutritionists. It reduces the body's need for oxygen, provides more available oxygen for mother and baby. Strengthens the circulatory system and helps to prevent miscarriage. D-alpha is natural. Synthetic does not work, DL-alpha tocopherol is synthetic.

Grains: When using grains be sure to eat a lot of fresh green vegetables. This prevents the calcium in the body from leaching out. Buckwheat is rich in magnesium, protein, providing the synthesis for oxidation of carbohydrates. Magnesium helps to prevent toxemia in pregnancy. Red meat can cause toxemia, so it would be better to substitute grains for meat. Whole grains include the bran and the germ which are full of nutrients. Contains B vitamins, vitamin E and iron. Helps eliminate constipation.

Heartburn: Papaya mint tea, ginger, alfalfa. Eat more food with B vitamins such as wheat germ and yogurt. Eat papaya tablets with meals. Eat smaller meals and eat slowly.

Iron: Builds the blood; essential for building the baby's liver. Eat cooked cereals, grains, raisins, apricots, prunes, molasses, brewers yeast, sunflower seeds, sesame seeds, kelp, egg yolks dulse and dry beans. Extra rich iron is found in dandelion and yellow dock, alfalfa, and liquid chlorophyll.

Lentils: Sprout before cooking, increases the nutrients.

Minerals: Very essential during pregnancy. Aluminum can leach out zinc. Even one mineral lacking in the body can cause birth defects.

Millet: Rich in protein, easy to digest. Use with vegetables, sesame and sunflower seeds.

Nausea: Eat smaller, more frequent meals for this prevents the blood sugar level from fluctuating. Eat protein before bed--sunflower seeds, ginger and papaya mint help in nausea. Low magnesium levels have been associated with nausea and vomiting. Blend papaya powder in milk for better assimilation. For severe nausea use vitamin E oil in rectum.

Protein: Very important, vegetable source is best. Use brown rice, buckwheat, millet, beans, grains, seeds and nuts.

Pumpkin Seeds: Rich in zinc and iron. The zinc can help prevent stretch marks.

Sesame Seeds: Rich source of methionine and other amino acids which are usually lacking in vegetables and grains. Use sesame seed milk.

Smoking: Avoid at all times, especially during pregnancy. The carbon monoxide prevents the intake of oxygen in the fetus and could cause birth defects. Increases the risk of miscarriage, fetal death or death soon after birth. Can cause stunted growth and birth weight and hyperactivity in children.

Sprouts: When using pure water to sprout it is one of the most uncontaminated, untreated foods that are available. Sprouting enhances the high nutritional value. The vitamins and minerals in sprouts are utilized more efficiently in the body. Mung and lentil sprouts provide balanced amino acids. Alfalfa: high calcium to phosphorus balance.

Stress: Pregnant women need a calm environment and emotional support. Studies have shown that emotional stress in pregnancy during the first trimester is capable of causing damage to the biological quality of the body. It alters the chemistry of the body. Exercise helps in stress; it helps use up the adrenaline that has assimilated during stress. Walking is good, relaxation is essential, at least a half hour of quiet time during the day. During stress take high doses of vitamin C (5,000 mg. per day). Protein is used up during stress. Use plant protein, for meat will put more stress on the body. Double B vitamins should be taken under stress. Alfalfa, brewers yeast, and wheat germ are effective foods. When using brewers yeast, is should be used with added calcium and magnesium.

Sugar: Excess absorbs quickly into the bloodstream and can affect the proper growth of the fetus. Sugar robs the body of nutrients.

Sweet Potatoes: Bake in the oven and when craving sweets use instead of white sugar products. Rich in vitamin A and C and minerals.

Vegetables: Eat a lot, for the more you eat the better. As much raw food as possible. Use a lot of green leafy vegetables such as watercress and leaf lettuce.

Zinc: Essential for vitamin A to be released from the liver. Necessary for proper growth of baby. Heals stretch marks and cuts.

6

INFANTS

Infants are totally dependent on the parent's knowledge of nutrition for their health and well-being. We are seeing babies born with physical and mental defects which has doubled in the last twenty years. We are witnessing babies born with cancer, crippling bone disease, arthritis, deformed bodies and many other disease. These have been traced to the inadequate diet of the mother deficient in the basic trace elements--especially minerals like iodine; and amino acids (building blocks of protein). The problem increases in those who consume alcohol and tobacco.

Nutritional deficiencies can permanently damage an infant's mental as well as physical development. The diet of infants has long lasting effect on their bodies for health or sickness. The infants who are already born with problems need nutritional supplements more than any other time in their lives. Proper food for the infants has a far reaching effect on the body for many years of its life, and will produce healthy bodies with an efficient immune system, strong nervous system and strong bones and teeth. The nervous system develops rapidly as the child obtains milk sugar. Lactose plays an important part on the myelination (the coating protection) of the nerves. Lactose is broken down into glucose and galactose. Galactose is vital for the myelination development, and cannot be found in any sugar other than lactose and breast milk and is the only known source of this lactose. Many nervous disorders could be avoided if babies could obtain the lactose for proper development of the nervous system. A well nourished baby will sleep well, wake up alert and with an appetite, satisfied with the feeding and will have a happy disposition.

The best protection and nourishment a mother can give her newborn is to nurse her baby. Many doctors now encourage mothers to nurse their babies, pointing out that mother's milk contains up to six times as much vitamin E as cow's milk and almost twice as much selenium (both immune protection supplements). The first few days are important for breast feeding. The mother secretes a clear yellow liquid called colostrum, which is high in protein and certain vitamins and minerals and lower in milk sugar and fat. Colostrum contains antibodies that protect the baby from infections that you will never find in commercial formulas. Colostrum protects against some of the most dangerous bacteria such as E. Colic which accounts for about 80 percent of cases of meningitis of the newborn. It protects against allergies. Breast fed infants have one half the incidence of inner ear infections, one fifth the incidence of respiratory infections, and two and one half times less digestive upsets than bottle-fed babies.

Breast milk can provide most of the baby's nutritional requirements during the first year of life. Even though solid foods are introduced around six months they cannot provide sufficient amounts to satisfy nutrient needs. The protein in mother's milk contains all the right amino acids, and is easier to digest. The iron in mother's milk is absorbed readily into the body.

Mother's milk contains beta-lactose in larger amounts than in cow's milk and is capable of producing a pure bacillus bifidus flora and maintaining it. This friendly bacteria produces B vitamin and lactic acid in mother's milk and is essential for the absorption of minerals into the blood. Anyone who believes that cow's milk is as good as mother's milk has not studied the facts.

Some of our processed baby formulas are manufactured by drug companies. Many nutritional doctors consider formula to be baby's first junk food and drug. Sweetened foods given to babies are linked to obesity, diabetes, diverticula disease and colon cancer. In 1950 thousands of parents in the United States were very concerned when their newborn babies went into convulsions without any explanation. One doctor noticed that these convulsions stopped when one infant's formula was changed. The company who manufactured the infant formula had forgotten to add vitamin B6 in their formula. It is frightening when we realize errors in industrial formulated baby formulas can cause illness as well as deficiency in nutritional value.

Cow's milk has too much protein and salt for human baby's system, and it puts a strain on their kidneys. The casein content of cow's milk helps build the bone structure of the baby calf, and is 300 times more potent than that in mother's milk. The cow's milk is intended to double the weight of the calf in 6 to 8 weeks. Infants require 6 to 7 months to double their body weight.

Low fat milk is not any better for babies, and many doctors call it a myth that it is better than whole milk. Lowfat milk is deficient in vitamins C, E and iron. It lacks essential fatty acids such as linoleic acid which is a vital nutrient for proper infant growth and central nervous system development.

Nutrients of breast fed babies depend on the mother's diet. If she eats a lot of junk food, that will be the quality of her milk. The baby will receive its nourishment from whatever the mother eats. Vitamin C and D are usually needed to supplement the breast fed baby. Vitamin C is needed every day and is vital in maintaining a healthy immune system. Some doctors feel that crib death could be eliminated with vitamin C supplementation to babies. Vitamin D supplement is also needed daily, especially when baby cannot get enough sunlight. Very few foods contain vitamin D. It is found in liver, egg yolks, and fresh liver oils.

When babies show increased appetite the mother needs to let her baby nurse more frequently instead of shoving cereal down its throat. The mother's milk will increase if the mother will add brewers yeast, blessed thistle, alfalfa, red raspberry and marshmallow to her diet. This will enhance rich milk for the baby.

Bottle Fed Babies

If it is impossible to nurse your baby, then supplements are essential. Bottle-fed babies need vitamins A, C, D; minerals such as iodine, iron, manganese and lecithin, and other essential nutrients such as lactic acid. Synthetic vitamin D which is found in infant formula has the ability to bind magnesium and to carry it out of the body. Magnesium deficiency could contribute to heart failure, interfere with nerve relay transmission and improper conduction of electrochemical impulses and lead to sleep apnea (cessation of breathing during sleep). Autopsy proves SIDS infants are low in magnesium. Synthetic vitamin D-2 is used in baby formula, children's breakfast cereals, and pasteurized and homogenized milk.

Crib death is more prevalent during the winter months, when we get less vitamin D from sunshine. All babies should have supplements of vitamin D, the natural kind. Cod liver oil is excellent to add to the babies diet. When using formulas from metal cans, remember that milk is slightly acid and can leach out the aluminum and cadmium. Fluoride in drinking water can create allergies in babies. We will discuss baby formulas and feeding babies later on.

Special Dietary Helps

Vitamin A: Infants need extra vitamin A, especially after the first three months. Vitamin A is reduced when infections are present, more is needed to produce antibodies to fight infections. Twins need more than single births.

Allergies: Introducing cereals as baby's first solid food can be a mistake. It can cause allergies because of improper digestion. Until the baby has teeth and has learned the chewing process and can ensalivate grains the proper enzyme for digestion is not present. Waiting until at least a year for cereals has shown that children would have almost no allergies, mucus, ear infections, colic, skin rashes and colds or other illnesses. It would help avoid assimilation and digestion problems later in life.

Asthma: Take Vitamins, A, C and D to strengthen the immune system. Mineral supplement, especially iodine found in kelp. Digestion problems are involved with lung problems. Adding papaya to babies diet would be beneficial. Allergies in baby's can cause asthma. Causes of asthma are malnutrition and irritated nerves. The nervous system should be built up by using catnip, tincture of lobelia, chamomile, comfrey, fenugreek, and a combination of herbs containing chickweed, comfrey, marshmallow and mullein. Fruits and vegetable should be the main diet, if the child is over six months of age and is bottle fed. For acute attacks of asthma, put a few drops of lobelia extract under the tongue, as well as rub it on the spine of the baby. Anti-spasmodic extract rubbed on the chest and back will also help.

Cadmium and Lead: They both interfere with the brain's neurotransmiters. Lead deposits in the brain causes brain damage, retardation. Metal poisoning contributes to criminal behavior, hyperactive children, bone ailments, depression, irritability and anger. Many babies are born with large amounts of lead and cadmium and this puts a stress on the nervous system. These toxic metals accumulate in small bodies.

The big danger of toxic metals is it displaces essential trace minerals, disrupting the body's metabolism and upsetting the chemical balance of the body. Toxic metals suppress the immune system and some have cancer causing elements.

Protection: B-complex and lecithin protect the nerve sheaths. Sulphur herbs such as garlic, onion, (make garlic & onion water), alfalfa (liquid chlorophyll), comfrey (small amounts in water), dandelion, kelp and lobelia help to protect the body. Zinc displaces lead and cadmium. Vitamin C with bioflavonoids are a natural chelation to metals. Kelp attaches itself to any lead and carries it harmlessly out of the system. Calcium penetrates the bones and slowly displaces lead. It prevents accumulation of lead in the tissues. Pectin (found in apples) removes lead. Cod liver oil helps inhibit the toxic build-up of cadmium.

Calcium: Calcium and magnesium deficiencies are associated with restlessness and constantly moving behavior. Low calcium is associated with difficulty falling asleep. Fevers from teething are common when there is not enough calcium available to help the teeth erupt. The body is trying to compensate by pulling calcium from the body wherever it can and causing disruption of the chemicals in the system. Giving the baby extra organic calcium along with vitamin A and D will help the teeth come through properly.

Colic: Colic in babies usually lasts from two to six weeks. Bottle fed babies have it more often. Nursing mothers should watch what they eat. Offending foods are beans, cabbage, garlic, onions, chocolate, tuna, eggs, corn and wheat. Catnip tea helps to relieve colic. Fennel and peppermint tea are also good. Enemas can give immediate relief. Bottle fed babies need more vitamin C, and B-complex vitamins, brewers yeast would help. Changing formulas have helped some babies with severe colic.

Constipation: Breast fed babies are seldom constipated. Bottle-fed babies are found to be constipated often. Cow's milk and the sugar used in formulas are most likely the cause. Using blackstrap molasses instead of sugar in formulas will help. Using the juice from stewed prunes and add to pure water will also help. Small amounts of cascara sagrada and ginger can be given to help regulate the infants bowels.

Vitamin C: Infants need a supplement of vitamin C daily along with bioflavonoids. It helps to detoxify substances. Nicotine from cigarettes prevents vitamin C from doing its job, the C is used up in detoxifying the nicotine from the system. Smoking around babies is very harmful. Vitamin C helps iron to be absorbed. It makes uric acid to resist bacterial infection. Helps build resistance to colds and infections. Maintains healthy bones and joints. Pollutants, aspirins, as well as other medications cause a loss of vitamin C.

Cuddling: Newborn babies are much more sensitive to their surroundings than some have supposed. Cuddling helps to satisfy the baby's early need for security and love.

Deficiencies: Children are most likely to be deficient in vitamins A, C, calcium and iron. Iron foods are sunflower seeds (made into milk), raisins (soaked and use the liquid), blackstrap molasses (added to the formula), dried apricots (soaked and added to juices). Calcium foods--Sesame seeds (made into milk), carrot juice (high in A and calcium) and alfalfa (make into a green drink and strain, use in juices).

Diaper Rash: Grind comfrey and golden seal and make a paste with aloe vera juice. Vitamins A and E are good. Corn starch to keep the rash dry.

Diarrhea: Diarrhea could be a mild intestinal infection, or something the mother ate which the baby does not tolerate. Mild diarrhea is common in young infants. Bottle-fed babies can get diarrhea from excess sugar in the formula, and also the lack of unsaturated fats in artificial formulas. Nursing mothers should add B-vitamins to their diet. Bottle fed babies can have brewers yeast added to their formula. Slippery Elm is very good for diarrhea. Carob powder, lemon in pure water, or barley water with a pinch of ginger will help relieve diarrhea.

Dry Skin: Olive oil, vitamin A and E, almond oil and aloe vera.

Earache: Keep babies' feet warm. The nerve endings in the bottom of the feet are sensitive to changes in temperature. Garlic oil in each ear, even though one ear is hurting. Garlic oil capsule in rectum. Mullein oil is very good to put in both ears; it helps stop the pain. Lobelia extract is also good for earaches. Bottle-fed babies should not be fed lying down, for the milk can back up into the ears and provide a breeding place for germs and cause infections.

Eyesight: Vitamin A is very important to give to infants. It is essential for good eyesight. Do not give babies salt; it can interfere with the eye development. Too much sugar leaches out the calcium from the body and can affect the veins of the eyes. Sunshine is very important for eye health. Carrot juice is a natural way to obtain high amounts of vitamin A and calcium, it contains more easily assimilated calcium than cow's milk. A very necessary food for infants. Plugged eye ducts usually correct themselves. Cleansing with pure water and massaging the area will sometimes help.

Fever: Fever helps the immune system. It causes the white cells (the infection fighters) to move rapidly to the infection site where they combat the problem. Antibodies increase in number and stop the microorganisms. Fever improves the effects of interferon, a chemical which stops the spread of viruses. Herb teas reduce fevers, provide nutrients and induce perspiration. Chamomile, catnip, slippery elm, red raspberry or spearmint tea are very helpful. Lemon juice, vitamin C powder in pure water, liquid chlorophyll or fruit juice about 30 minutes before before breast feeding. An enema if the fever is prolonged.

Hyperactivity: Babies can suffer from hyperactivity. They can be born with it. Keep baby away from sweets, and remember they are in artificial formulas. They lead to an excess of glucose in the blood within a half hour. Keep them away from artificial coloring, which can even be in vitamin preparations. B-complex in water or juice is very calming to the nerves. Organic calcium supplements are also good for the nerves. Minerals are very important; zinc alone is responsible for other nutrient's assimilation. Vitamin A and D are necessary. The central nervous system is involved in all allergic reactions.

Immunization: Parents have the right to accept or reject vaccinations for their children. Infants are born with protection of viral or bacterial infections and they will continue to receive it from their mother's milk. A natural immunization results when the body is exposed to various disease and a resistance is high or low. Building the immune system with vitamin A, C, B-complex vitamins and minerals will help protect the baby. Immunization is an artificial approach and is supposed to prevent diseases in the future. There is no concrete evidence that vaccinations are effective as a preventive measure. It is taken from sick cows, and can cause mental damage from the cowpox virus to the brain. It is felt by some doctors that Infant Death Syndrome may be due to poisons ingested into the body. Viruses are always present in the body. A rundown body or poorly nourished, leaves it wide open for virus attacks. It is felt that meningitis could be a side-effect of the smallpox vaccine. It you decide on vaccinating your baby, avoid having it done during the summer or hot weather. Clean the body with herbal laxatives. Give the baby high amounts of vitamin A and C to protect the immune system.

Jaundice: Jaundice is an indication that the liver and gallbladder need a boost. Lemon juice in water will help clean the liver. A few drops of vitamin E in the baby's mouth after nursing will help.

Reye's Syndrome: Doctors are recommending that aspirin not be given to children suffering from flu or chicken pox symptoms. Reye's Syndrome is an acute illness of children characterized by an encephalitic-like state with fever, vomiting, disturbances of consciousness progressing to coma or convulsion. Build the babies' immune system to prevent Reye's Syndrome by keeping sweets away, supplement with vitamin A, C with bioflavonoids, and vitamin D. Minerals should also be given.

SIDS: Sudden Infant Death Syndrome is the leading

cause of death in American babies more than a week old. Parents put an apparently healthy baby to bed at night and find it dead in the morning. There are many theories, and many investigations seeking to identify high-risk infants. Each years thousands of babies between 4 weeks and 7 months of age die in their sleep.

Many health-minded doctors feel that supplying the baby with supplements such as vitamin A (cod liver oil), with D, vitamin C (the liquid form is easy for babies), vitamin E, squeezed in the mouth after feeding and supplements such as brewers yeast and blackstrap molasses help provide minerals to build up the baby's immune system. Iron, selenium and magnesium have been found lacking in babies who have died from crib deaths.

Researchers at St. John's University in New York found evidence to suggest SIDS is caused by allergic reaction in infants who have deficiencies in their immune system. The babies lack the ability to combat allergies in such common items as cow's milk, household dust or fungal spores in the air, said Constantine J. Efthymiou, a professor of biological sciences at St. John's (*Health Fact News*, May 1982).

Slippery Elm:
Added to babies formula, will help the milk to digest. The powder can be made into a gruel or beverage and is a bland nutritive food for babies. The gruel is a valuable remedy in cases of weakness, stomach inflammations, lung hemorrhage and pulmonary complaints.

Teething: Restless, crying babies who are teething need more calcium and vitamin D. Add powdered calcium and vitamin C to juice. Weak warm catnip tea will help the nerves and calm the baby. Rubbing the gums with lobelia extract will help. Rubbing with clove oil and aloe vera juice will also help. Sore gums can be rubbed with thick honey to which a pinch of salt has been added. Honey with oil of chamomile, peppermint or fennel will help.

Thrush: Clean the mouth with fresh lemon water. Oil of garlic can be put in the mouth as well as spread on the baby's bottom. Acidophilus is very important in healing and discouraging thrush. If the mother is nursing she should take acidophilus as well as yogurt. Acidophilus can be rubbed inside the babies mouth, and a capsule can be inserted up the rectum. High sugar diets of mother and formulas high in refined sugars encourage thrush. The nursing mother needs more B vitamins and bottle fed babies need supplements of brewers yeast and molasses.

Vomiting: An infant who is vomiting should be given fluids often because a baby can dehydrate very quickly. If the mother is nursing she should nurse more often and during a short period so the baby can have time to make sure the milk stays down. A few drops of lobelia tincture in the mouth will help to relax the stomach. Pure water often will also help. Liquid chlorophyll in pure water is helpful.

Worms: Worms as well as parasites can effect babies because they put everything in their mouths. Mother's milk is a natural cleanser. A few drops of black walnut extract will help. Ringworm can be treated with a pinch of black walnut and golden seal moistened with aloe vera and applied to the skin. For Impetigo, use black walnut. Black walnut contains iodine which is a strong antiseptic.

Nourishing Infant Formulas

15 ounces barley water
10 ounces milk (goat or cow)
1 tsp pure maple syrup
1 to 3 crushed papaya tablets

To make barley water, put one cup barley in cheese cloth and tie loosely in 2 quarts pure water. Use pure water for the chlorine content, could cause allergies. Boil for 6 hours, add more water, and boil down to 15 ounces of barley water.

Almond and Sesame Milk Formula

1 cup chopped almonds
1/2 cup sesame seeds
1 quart pure water
1 tsp pure maple syrup

Soak the almonds and seeds overnight in the refrigerator. Blend for 3 minutes at high speed and strain.

Almonds and Cashew Milk Formula

Use raw nuts and seeds

1/2 C. almonds
1/2 C. cashews
1/4 C. raisins
1 T molasses
1/2 tsp slippery elm powder
1 quart of pure water

Soak all together overnight. Blend and strain.

Baby's First Foods
6 months to 1 year

Breast milk should be the most important food along with vitamin A, D and C. At 6 months liquid vitamin and mineral supplements may be added. Gradually add foods one at a time to make certain baby does not develop any allergies.

Ripe avocado with ripe mashed bananas is a wonderful first food for the infant. Steam carrots and blend and dilute with nut or seed milk. Squash, zucchini or summer squash blended. Baked winter squash can also be diluted with almond milk or sesame milk. Green beans, steamed and blended. Fruits, scraped apples or ripe pears are excellent for babies. Juices are very good. Carrot juice, strained and diluted. Try to feed fruit and vegetables at different times to avoid any food combination allergies. After feeding the baby wait at least 30 minutes to nurse. This gives time for the food to digest before liquids are eaten, which can cause intestinal problems such as gas.

7

SINGLE HERBS

Alfalfa
(Medicago sativa)
Parts Used: Leaves and flowers

Specific Uses: Stomach and blood; benefits bladder and prostate; helps in chemical imbalance; rich in trace minerals lacking in the average American diet; cleans blood in toxemia in pregnancy; neutralizes uric acid for arthritis, bursitis, etc.; useful to prevent cholesterol accumulation in the veins; cleans, builds and strengthens the body; saponin properties clean deep in the cells and bind serum/cholesterol, radioactive deposits and toxins in the system for elimination; eight digestive enzymes in alfalfa provide better digestion and assimilation; alkaloid in the leaves strengthens the central nervous system; rebuilds decayed teeth; beneficial effect on pituitary gland; relieves pain and inflammation.

Vitamin and Mineral Content: Rich in chlorophyll, protein, vitamin A, E, K, D, B6 and U. Also rich in calcium and trace minerals. Contains high amounts of phosphorus, iron, potassium, chlorine, sodium, silicon, magnesium B1, B2 nd B12. Has 8 of the essential amino acids.

Ailments
Acid Stomach, Alcoholism, *Allergies, Anemia*, Appendicitis (chronic), *Appetite Stimulant, Arthritis,* Cancer, Cholesterol Reducer, Cramps, Diabetes, Digestion, *Diuretic (mild), Fatigue (mental and physical),* Fever, *Glands, Gout, Hemorrhages,* high Blood Pressure, Jaundice, *Kidney Cleanser,* Lactation (quantity and quality), *Radiation Damage, Teeth, Tonic,* Toxemia, *Ulcers,* Urinary Problems, *Vitamin and Mineral Deficiency.*

Aloe Vera
(Aloe ssp.)
parts Used: Fresh Juice or Powdered

Specific Uses: Skin, stomach and colon; cleans, heals, soothes and relieves pain on contact; contains salicyclic acid and magnesium which work together directly on burns as an aspirin-like analgesic effect; cleans, builds, and strengthens the system; glycoside almoin stimulates colon cleanse and eliminates toxins; the uronic acid cleans toxic materials from the skin area to prevent harmful irritations; helps heal throat problems, hiatal hernia and intestinal problems; relieves itching in shingles and chicken pox.

Vitamin and Mineral Content: High in vitamin C and selenium. Contains moderate amounts of sodium, vitamin A and niacin. Has small amounts of calcium, magnesium, phosphorus, potassium, iron, zinc, manganese and B-complex. Contains trace amounts of copper, B2 and lecithin.

Ailments
Abrasions, Acne, Anemia, Arthritis, Bites, *Burns,*
Colitis, Constipation, *Deodorant, Digestion,* Fever,
Hair (stimulant), Heartburn, *Hemorrhoids, Hiatal
Hernia, Insect Bites,* Leg Ulcers, Liver Problems,
Menopause, Obesity, Poison Ivy and Oak, Psoriasis,
Radiation Burns, Ringworm, *Scalds, Scar Tissues,*
Sores, Sunburn, Tapeworm, Tuberculosis, Tumors,
Wrinkling of Skin, Ulcered Sores, Ulcers, Vaginitis,
Worms, Wounds.

Barberry
(Berberis vulgaris)
Parts Used: Root Bark

Specific Uses: Liver, spleen digestive system, blood;
special cleansing effect on the body--especially the
stomach and bowels; contains saponin, recognized as
a deep cleansing agent, and an alkaloid berberine
which has the ability to kill parasites; reduces blood
pressure; excellent cancer herb.

Vitamin and Mineral Content: High in calcium,
iron, chlorine and sulphur. Also high in the following
B vitamins: B1, B2, pantothenic acid, niacin, biotin,
choline and folic acid.

Ailments
Acne, Arthritis, Boils, Blood Pressure (lowers), *Blood
Purifier,* Cancer, Colitis, Constipation, *Diarrhea,*
Dysentery, Dyspepsia, Fevers, *Gall Bladder,* Gum
Diseases, Hemorrhages, *Indigestion, Jaundice,*
Laxative, *Liver Problems,* Parasites, Polyps,
Pyorrhea, Spleen Problems, *Throat (sore),* Ulcers.

Bayberry
(Myrica cerifera)
Parts Used: Root Bark

Specific Uses: Skin, circulation, stomach and intestines; aids in digestion, nutrition and building the blood; it has cleansing properties--helps get rid of toxic mucus and growths in female tract; builds and strengthens the system; contains strong germicidal properties which destroy harmful bacteria; tones and promotes glandular activity while cleansing; stops profuse menstruation and menstrual cramps; effective when combined with ginger and capsicum to fight colds and flu; excellent gargle for sore throats and bleeding gums; helps fight bronchopulmonary diseases, sinuses and adenoid problems.

Vitamin and Mineral Content: Very high in vitamin C and calcium. Contains moderate amounts of phosphorus, potassium and zinc. Contains trace amounts of niacin, B1, B2, vitamin A, sodium, chlorine, magnesium, manganese and silicon.

Ailments
Asthma, Bleeding, Bleeding Gums, Boils, Bronchitis, Canker Sores, Carbuncles, Catarrh, *Cholera,* Colitis, *Diarrhea, Dysentery,* Dyspepsia, Epilepsy, Eyes, Fever, Flu, Gangrenous Sores, Gargle, *Glands, Goiter,* Headaches, hemorrhoids, *Indigestion, Infections, Jaundice,* Leucorrhea, *Liver Problems*, Lumbago, Lungs, *Menstrual Bleeding, Scrofula,* Sluggishness, Scurvy, Syphilis, Throat (sore and ulcerated), Thrush, Thyroid, Ulcers *Uterine Hemorrhage,* Uterus (prolapsed).

Bilberry
(Vaccinium myrtillus)
Parts Used: Fruit

Specific Uses: The eyes, it rebuilds retina purple pigments in the eyes; used effectively for night vision and light sensitive eyes; beneficial as a nutritive herb; rich in manganese which improves eyesight; people have been found to benefit within a few months for night blindness when using bilberry.

Vitamin and Mineral content: It is rich in manganese, phosphorus, iron and zinc. Contains moderate amounts of magnesium, potassium and selenium. Contains trace amounts of calcium, sodium and silicon.

Ailments
Eyes, Immune System, Blood Vessels, Kidney Problems, Light Sensitive Eyes, *Night Blindness*, Varicose Veins.

Black Cohosh
(Cimicifuga racemosa)
Parts Used: Root

Specific Uses: Uterus, nerves, lungs, and heart; used in last weeks of pregnancy to strengthen and stimulate uterine contractions in childbirth; acts directly on the spinal nerves as a relaxing nervine; loosens and expels mucus from the bronchial tubes; equalizes blood circulation; stimulates natural estrogen production and many women benefit from its use during menopause instead of resorting to estrogen supplements; effective in balancing hormones.

Vitamin and Mineral Content: Rich in phosphorus, calcium, and is high in selenium. Contains moderate amounts of magnesium, potassium and iron. Also has moderate amounts of vitamin K and F (fatty acids), Contains small amounts of sodium, silicon, manganese, zinc, vitamin A, C, niacin, B1 and B2 and a trace of sulphur.

Ailments
Arthritis, *Asthma*, Bites (insect and snake), *Bronchitis*, Childbirth, Cholera, Convulsions, Coughs, Cramps, *Epilepsy*, Headaches, Heart Stimulant, *High Blood Pressure, Hormone Balance*, Hot Flashes, Hysteria, Insomnia, Kidney Problems, Liver Problems, Lumbago, *Lungs, Menopause, Menstrual Problems*, Nervous Disorders, Neuralgia, Pain, Rheumatism, Skin Problems, Smallpox, *St. Virus Dance, Tuberculosis*, Uterine Problems, *Whooping Cough*.

Black Walnut
(Juglans nigra)
Parts Used: Hulls and Leaves

Specific Uses: Blood, intestines, and nerves; benefits from rich organic iodine and tannins which contain antiseptic properties; oxygenating abilities burn up excess toxins and fatty materials; helps to regulate blood sugar levels; used for herpes and impetigo; contains natural fluoride--removes plaque and restores tooth enamel; externally, heals athletes foot; counteracts hemorrhoidal bleeding in colon.

Vitamin and Mineral Content: It is high in manganese, selenium, potassium, iodine and B15. It contains moderate amounts of iron and sodium.

Small amounts of calcium, magnesium, phosphorus, silicon, chlorine, phosphorus, and B1. It contains small amounts of vitamin A, C, niacin, B2, B6, and P, the bioflavonoids.

Ailments
Abscesses, Acne, Antiperspirant, *Antiseptic (external)*, Boils, Cancer, Carbuncles, Colitis, Diphtheria, Eczema, Electrical Shock, Eye Diseases, Fevers, Gargle, Hemorrhoids, Infections, *Lactation (stops)*, Liver, Lupus, Mouthsores, *Parasites (internal)*, Poison Ivy, *Rashes, (skin, Ringworm)*, Scrofula, Tonsillitis, Tuberculosis, Tumors, Ulcers (internal), Uterus (prolapsed), Varicose Veins, *Worms*, Wounds.

Blessed Thistle
(Cnicus benedictus)
Parts Used: The Herb

Specific Uses: Digestion, heart, blood, mammary glands and uterus; balances hormones; increases mother's milk; good for menopause and female problems; combined with warm chamomile tea helps bring quick relief from menstrual cramps; helpful for young girls in puberty; takes oxygen to brain and helps circulation (disease preventative); strengthens memory, heart, and lungs; rids system of tumors.

Vitamin and Mineral Content: Rich in vitamin A, potassium, and selenium. Moderate amounts of B complex, magnesium, phosphorus, sodium and iron. Small amounts of vitamin C, niacin and zinc.

Ailments
Arthritis, Birth Control, *Blood Circulation, Blood Purifier,* Cancer, Constipation, Cramps, Digestion, Dropsy, Fevers, *Gallbladder,* Gas, *Headaches, Heart (strengthens), Hormones (balances),* Jaundice, Kidneys, *Lactation,* Leucorrhea, *Liver Ailments, Lungs (strengthens),* Memory, *Menstrual Problems,* Respiratory Infections, Senility, Spleen, Worms.

Blue Cohosh
(Caulophyllum thalictroides)
Parts Used: Root

Specific Uses: Uterus, nerves, joints (muscular pain), urinary tract; cleanses, builds and helps to sustain health; strengthens uterus for easier delivery when the body is ready; useful for uterine disorders; contains anti-bacterial properties to calm nerves and relieve muscular pain; regulates menstruation; helps heart palpitations; soothes.

Vitamin and Mineral Content: Rich in iron. High in manganese, selenium, and vitamin E. Contains moderate amounts of calcium, magnesium, phosphorus, potassium, silicon, vitamin B1 and B2. Small amounts of vitamin A, C, niacin, sodium and chlorine, and zinc.

Ailments
Ague, Bladder Infections, Colic, Convulsions, *Cramps,* Diabetes, Dropsy, *Epilespy,* Fits, High Blood Pressure, *Labor (induces),* Leucorrhea, Menstruations (regulates), Muscular Cramps, *Nerves,* Neuralgia, Pregnancy Disorders, Spasms, *Uterine (chronic problems),* Vaginitis.

Blue Vervain
(Verbena officinalis)
Parts Used: The Herb

Specific Uses: Circulation, lungs, nerves, spleen, liver, and bowels; promotes sweating, relaxes nerves, soothes and allays fevers in virus colds; settles stomach; produces an overall relaxed well-being.

Vitamin and Mineral Content: Contains moderate amounts of vitamin C and E. Also calcium and manganese.

Ailments
Ague, *Asthma, Bladder, Bowels, Bronchitis,* Catarrh, *Colds, Colon, Consumption,* Congestion (throat and chest), *Convulsion, Coughs,* Diarrhea, Dysentery and Earaches, Epilepsy, Female Problems, *Fevers,* Gallstones, Headaches, *Insomnia,* Kidney Problems Menstrual Problems, Mucus, Nerves, Pneumonia, Skin Diseases, Sores, Spleen, *Stomach (settles),* Worms.

Boneset
(Eupatorium perfoliatum)
Parts Used: Their Herb

Specific Uses: Stomach, liver, intestines and circulation; considered the best remedy for relief of flu symptoms--to induce sweating and to combat muscular pains, colds and fevers take warm--to reduce chills and shakes of a fever take cool; cleans the stomach, liver, and intestines of toxins and eliminates them from the body.

Vitamin and Mineral Content: Contains moderate amounts of vitamin C, calcium, vitamin B-complex, magnesium and potassium.

Ailments
Bronchitis, Catarrh, *Chills, Colds, Fever Prevention, Fevers (all kinds), Flu,* Jaundice, Liver Disorders, Malaria, Measles, Mumps, Pneumonia, Rheumatism (muscular), Rocky Mountain Spotted Fever, Scarlet Fever, Throat (sore), Tonic, *Typhoid Fever,* Worms, *Yellow Fever.*

Buchu
(Barosma betulina)
Parts Used: Leaves

Specific Uses: Bladder and kidneys; considered one of the best herbs for the urinary tract; contains antiseptic properties with camphor like qualities--its active part of the oil; great for painful urination and bladder inflammations; soothes the enlargement of the prostate gland and irritation of the urethral membrane.

Vitamin and Mineral Content: Rich in calcium, potassium and sodium. High amounts of phosphorus, iron, zinc, selenium, manganese. Moderate amounts of magnesium and small amounts of silicon.

Ailments
Bed Wetting, Bladder, Catarrh, Cancer, Cystitis, Diabetes (first stages), Dropsy, Gallstones, *Kidney Problems, Nephritis, Prostate Problems,* Rheumatism, *Urethritis,* Yeast Infections.

Buckthorn
(Rhamnus catharticus)
Parts Used: Bark and Berries

Specific Uses: Liver, gallbladder, blood and intestines; stimulating effect on the bile; positive effect on conditions of the liver, gallbladder and lower bowels; does not gripe and keeps the bowels regular without irritation.

Vitamin and Mineral Content: Contains moderate amounts of calcium, phosphorus, and potassium, small amounts of sodium and chlorine. Trace amounts of magnesium, iron, manganese, copper and zinc.

Ailments
Appendicitis, *Bleeding, Bowels, Constipation (chronic),* Dropsy, *Fevers, Gallstones,* Gout, Hemorrhoids, Itching, *Lead Poisoning, Liver,* Parasites, Rheumatism, Skin Diseases, Warts (external), Worms.

Bugleweed
(Lycopus virginicus)
Parts Used: The Herb

Specific Uses: Respiratory, nervous system; irregular heartbeat; chronic inflammation of the lungs; overactive thyroid; nervous heart palpitation; eases irritating nervous coughs; use with yellow dock for lead poisoning.

Vitamin and Mineral Content: Bugleweed is a member of the mint family. Probably contains vitamin A and C. Also calcium, potassium and phosphorus.

Ailments
Asthma, Bleeding, Bronchitis, Colds, *Coughs,* Diabetes, Diarrhea, Dysentery, Fevers, Heart Palpitation, Hemorrhaging (pulmonary), *Indigestion (Nervous), Menstruation (excess),* Multiple Sclerosis, *Nerves,* Nosebleeds, *Pain,* Sores, Thyroid, Tuberculosis, Ulcers.

Burdock
(Arctium lappa)
Parts Used: Root

Specific Uses: Blood, kidneys and liver; considered one of best blood purifiers to eliminate uric acid and excess waste material; contains mucilage--with antifungal and anti-bacterial properties; soothes hypothalamus; aids the pituitary gland to help adjust hormone balance; relieves congestion of lymphatic system ;helps break down calcification in joints.

Vitamin and Mineral Content: Rich in vitamin C, iron and magnesium. Rich in inulin--a form of starch. High in phosphorus, potassium, sodium, silicon and B1. Moderate amounts of calcium selenium, manganese, vitamin A and P. Small amounts of vitamin E, niacin, B2 and PABA. Trace amounts of chlorine, sulphur, iodine and copper.

Ailments
Acne, Allergies, *Arthritis,* Asthma, *Blood Purifier,* Boils, Bronchitis, Canker Sore, Cancer, Dandruff, *Eczema,* Fevers, *Gout,* Hay Fever, Infections, *Kidney*

Problems, Leprosy, Liver Problems, Lumbago, Lungs, Nervousness, *Rheumatism, Skin Diseases,* Uterus (prolapsed), Wounds.

Butcher's Broom
(*Ruscus aculeatus*)
Parts Used: Root

Specific Uses: Circulation and urinary tract; effective in improving circulation to prevent post-operative thrombosis, varicose veins, phlebitis and hemorrhoids; prevents clotting of the blood by producing a diuretic effect; strengthens the blood vessels; also an herbal food to help keep the veins clean and healthy.

Vitamin and Mineral Content: High in iron, niacin, B1 and zinc. Moderate amounts of calcium, potassium, manganese, selenium and vitamin C. Small amounts of sodium, vitamin A and B2.

Ailments
Atherosclerosis, Brain (circulation), Circulation (increases), *Dropsy,* Headaches, Heavy Legs, *Hemorrhoids,* Leg Cramps, Menstrual Problems, *Phlebitis (vein inflammation), Thrombosis (blood clotting).*

Bee Pollen

An excellent anti-aging and energy supplement. It contains detoxifying and health building properties. It contains rich sources of vitamins, minerals, protein, amino acids, hormones, enzymes and fats. Every chemical substance needed to maintain life is present in bee pollen. It is a complete food. A very good supplement to build the immune system and provide energy for the body. It contains vitamins A, C, D, E and K--also contains lecithin, B vitamins and the rare plant source of B12. There are 22 amino acids and 27 minerals in bee pollen.

Bee Pollen has helped those with allergies and hay fever to build up immunity, starting with small doses. The bee pollen mixed with honey is used in Russia for treating hypertension, nervous and endocrine system complaints. Bee pollen improves appetite, normalizes activity of the intestines and increase fitness for work. It strengthen capillary walls; helps alleviates uremia--blood in urine, offset effects of drugs, pollutants; aids in radiation sickness; heals colitis and improves anemia.

Ailments
Alcoholism, *Allergies,* Anemia, *Asthma,* Blood Pressure (lowers) Cancer, Depression, Digestion, *Endurance, Energy, Exhaustion, Hay Fever,* Hypoglycemia, Liver disorders, *Longevity,* Prostate Disorders, *Vatility*

Capsicum or Cayenne
(Capsicum frutescens)
Parts Used: Fruit

Specific Uses: Heart, circulation, stomach, and kidneys; used as a crisis herb--a first aid remedy for most conditions; stops bleeding, heart attacks, strokes, colds, flu, low vitality, headaches, indigestion, depression and arthritis; powerful stimulant--circulation in the body is the key to healing; used with lobelia for tetanus and as a nervine.

Vitamin and Mineral Content: Rich in zinc. High in vitamin A, C, iron, calcium, potassium and rutin. Moderate amounts of vitamin G, magnesium, phosphorus, sulphur, and B-complex. Small amounts of sodium, and selenium.

Ailments
Malaria, *Arthritis, Bleeding*, Blood Cleanser, *Blood Pressure Equalizer*, Bronchitis, Bruises, Burns, Congestion, Chills, *Circulation, Diabetes,* Eyes, Fatigue, Fevers, Gas, *Heart, High Blood Pressure,* Infection, Jaundice, *Kidney Problems*, Lockjaw, Lung Problems, Mucus, Pancreas, Pyorrhea, *Rheumatism,* Shock Sprains (external), *Strokes*, Sunburns, Throat (sore), *Tumors, Ulcers*, Varicose Veins, Wounds.

Cascara Sagrada
(Rhamnus purshiana)
Parts Used: Bark

Specific Uses: Colon, stomach, liver, gallbladder and pancreas; considered one of the very best and safest laxatives in the herbal kingdom; antibiotic effect on harmful bacteria in the intestines; helps with insomnia, high blood pressure and digestive complaints; bitter principles stimulate the secretions of the entire digestive system; restores tone to the relaxed bowel for a beneficial permanent effect.

Vitamin and Mineral Content: Rich in calcium. Contains moderate amounts of potassium, phosphorus, selenium and vitamin A. Small amounts of sodium, chlorine, magnesium, iron, and niacin. Trace of manganese, silicon, vitamin C, B1, and B2.

Ailments

Catarrh, *Colon, Constipation,* Coughs, Croup, Digestion, Dyspepsia, *Gallbladder, Gallstones,* Gout, Hemorrhoids, High Blood Pressure, Indigestion, Insomnia, *Intestines,* Jaundice, *Liver Disorders,* Nerves, Pituitary, Spleen, Worms.

Calendula or Marigold
(Calendula officinalis)
Parts Used: Flowers

Specific Uses: Blood and skin; used internally as a warm infusion to treat fevers, ulcers, cramps and eruptive skin diseases (smallpox and measles); used externally for bee stings, skin disease, wounds, varicose veins; oil used for earaches--heals with speed and relieves inflammation both internal and external; good first aid remedy; snuff to discharge mucus from the nose; used as tincture applied to bruises and sprains.

Vitamin and Mineral Content: High in phosphorus. Contains vitamin A and C.

Ailments

Anemia, Blood Cleanser, Bronchitis, *Bruises (external),* Cancer, Colitis, Cramps, *Cuts (external),* Diarrhea, Ear Infections, Eye Infections, Fevers, Hepatitis, Jaundice, *Skin Diseases,* Sores (External), Toothache, Ulcers, Varicose Veins, Worms (expels), Wounds.

Catnip
(Nepeta cataria)
Parts Used: Their Herb

Specific Uses: Nerves and intestines; has calming effect on stomach cramps, spasms, gas and nervous disorders; essential oils act as expectorant in coughs, and cramps helps in digestion; great tonic to balance the body.

Vitamin and Mineral Content: Rich in iron and selenium. High in potassium, manganese, vitamin A and C. Moderate amounts of magnesium and phosphorus. Contains small amounts of calcium, sodium and silicon, and some B-complex.

Ailments
Anemia, Bronchitis (chronic), Circulation (improves), *Colds, Colic, Convulsions,* Coughs, Cramps (menstrual), *Diarrhea, Digestion,* Diseases (childhood), Drug Withdrawal, Fatigue, *Fevers, Flu, Gas,* Headaches (nervous), Hemorrhoids, Hiccups, Infertility, Insanity, Lung Congestion, Menstruation (suppressed), Miscarriage Preventive, Morning Sickness, Nicotine Withdrawal, *Nerves,* Pain, Restlessness, Shock, Skin, Sores (external), Spasms, Stress, Stomach Upset, Vomiting, Worms.

Chamomile
(Anthemis nobilis)
Parts Used: Flower

Specific Uses: Nerves, stomach, kidneys, liver, uterus and circulation; contains tryptophan, which works like a sedative in the body to induce natural sleep; useful as a steam inhalant for bronchial disorders; helps regulate menstrual flow and drug withdrawal.

Vitamin and Mineral Content: Contains high amounts of calcium and magnesium. Contains moderate amounts of potassium, phosphorus and manganese. Has small amounts of vitamin A, C, E and F, iron, some B-complex, selenium, silicon, pantothenic acid, and zinc.

Ailments
Air pollution, *Appetite Stimulant,* Asthma (steam inhalant), Bladder, *Bronchitis,* Catarrh, Childhood Diseases, Constipation, Colds, Coughs, *Cramps (menstrual),* Cramps (stomach), Diarrhea, Drug (withdrawal), Earache (compress), Eye (sore), *Fevers,* Gallstones, Gas, Headaches, *Hysteria,* Indigestion, *Insomnia,* Jaundice, Kidneys, Measles, *Menstrual (suppressant), Nervousness,* Pain Spasms, Stomach Upset, Teething, Throat (gargle), Tumors, Typhoid, Peptic Ulcers.

Chaparral
(Larrea tridentata)
Parts Used: Leaves and Stems

Specific Uses: Stomach, intestines, lungs, and has a general effect on the whole body; fights bacteria, viruses and parasites--internally and externally; saponins act as a natural "detergent" in cleansing the system of toxic impurities; contains an acid NDGA (nordihydroguaiaretic) which has the properties to convert fermentation process thought to be out of balance; best herbal antibiotic; has a definite cancer potential in decreasing tumor and leukemia; takes drugs out of system--especially LSD; rebuilds tissue.

Vitamin and Mineral Content: High in vitamin A, calcium and selenium. Contains moderate amounts of vitamin C, protein, magnesium, potassium, iron and manganese. Small amounts of phosphorus, sodium, zinc and B-complex vitamins.

Ailments
Aches, Acne, Allergies, *Arthritis,* Backaches (chronic), *Blood Purifier,* Boils, Bowels (lower), Bruises, Bursitis, *Cancer*, Cataracts, Colds, Cuts, Eczema, Eyes (strengthen), Hemorrhoids, Kidney Infection, *Leukemia*, Prostate, Psoriasis, Respiratory System, Rheumatism, Stomach Disorders, *Tumors*, Uterus (prolapsed), Venereal Disease, Wounds.

Chickweed
(Stellaria media)
Parts Used: The Whole Herb

Specific Uses: Blood, liver, lungs, kidneys and bladder; helps with youthful appearance and healthy mental attitude with its nutrients to feed and nourish the pineal and pituitary glands; mild but valuable herb to nourish and cleanse the system; helps dissolve plaque in blood vessels and fatty tumors; anti-cancer agent.

Vitamin and Mineral Content: Rich in iron, vitamin C and zinc. High amounts of calcium, magnesium, phosphorus, potassium, sodium, manganese, silicon. Moderate in B-complex and vitamin D.

Ailments
Appetite (decreases), Arteriosclerosis, Asthma, *Bleeding, Blood Purifier,* Bronchitis, Bruises, Bursitis, Cancer Preventive, Colitis, Constipation, *Convulsions,* Cramps, Eye Infections, Gas, Hemorrhoids, Lung Congestion, Mucus, *Obesity,* Pleurisy, *Skin Rashes,* Testicles (swollen), Tissues (inflamed), *Ulcers,* Water Retention, Wounds.

Comfrey
(Symphytum officinale)
Parts Used: Leaves and Roots

Specific Uses: Bones, skin, muscles, general effect on the whole body; cleans up dead tissues while healing; eliminates bloody urine; healing for respiratory system; suppresses bleeding; great cell proliferant or new cell grower on flesh and bones;

destroys amoebic-like bacteria as well as to prevent further growth; can dislodge mucus from inside lung chambers.

Vitamin and Mineral Content: Rich in vitamin A, C and trace minerals. High in protein, calcium, potassium, phosphorus, iron. Moderate amounts of magnesium, sulphur, and zinc. Contains eighteen amino acids. Small amounts of selenium and some B-complex vitamins as well as B12 (usually found only in animal protein).

Ailments
Allergies, *Anemia, Arthritis,* Asthma, Bladder, Bleeding, *Blood Cleanser, Boils, Bone breaks,* Bronchitis, *Bruises, Burns,* Bursitis, Cancer, Colds, Colitis, Coughs, Cramps, Diarrhea, Digestion, Emphysema, Eczema, Fatigue, *Fractures,* Gangrene, Gout, Hay Fever, Infections, Insect Bites, Kidney Stones, Leg Cramps, *Lungs,* Pain, Pleurisy, Pneumonia, Respiratory Problems, Sinusitis, Skin Problems, *Sores, Sprains,* Stomach Trouble, *Swelling,* Tonic, Tuberculosis.

Cornsilk
(Stigmata maidis)
Parts Used: Silky Tassels of Corn

Specific Uses: Kidneys, bladder and prostate; strong diuretic to promote urination; helps fight infections in the urethra, bladder, kidneys and prostate; rich in vitamin K; helps control bleeding--effective during childbirth to control bleeding as well as clean the urinary tract.

Vitamin and Mineral Content: High amounts of iron, silicon and vitamin K. Moderate amounts of magnesium, phosphorus, potassium and zinc. Small amounts of calcium, selenium, manganese, niacin, and B1. Trace amounts of sodium, vitamin A, C, and B2.

Ailments
Arteriosclerosis, Bed Wetting, *Bladder Infection,* Cholesterol, Cystitis, Dropsy, Gonorrhea, Heart Disease, High Blood Pressure, Inflammation, *Kidney Problems,* Obesity, Pain, Prostate Gland, Renal Inflammation, Scalding Urine, Uric Acid Buildup, Urinary Problems, Water Retention.

Damiana
(Turnera aphrodisiaca)
Parts Used: Leaves

Specific Uses: Reproductive organs, nerves and kidneys; small amounts act as a tonic to the nervous system; historically used to strengthen the male sexual system; contains properties to stimulate male hormone testosterone.

Vitamin and Mineral Content: High amounts of vitamin A, iron and niacin. Moderate amounts of magnesium, potassium, manganese and vitamin C. Small amounts of phosphorus, selenium, silicon, B1 and sodium. Trace amounts of zinc and B2.

Ailments
Brain Tonic, *Bronchitis,* Depression, Energy, *Emphysema*, Exhaustion, Female Problems, Frigidity, *Hormone Balance, Hot Flashes, Impotency, Infertility, Menopause,* Nerves, *Parkinson's Disease,*

Prostate, *Reproductive Organs, Sexual Stimulant,*
Weakness.

Dandelion
(Taraxacum officinale)
Parts Used: Leaves and Roots

Specific Uses: Liver, kidneys, gall bladder, stomach,
pancreas, intestines and blood; considered a nutritive
herb with medicinal benefits; soothes the digestive
tract and absorbs toxins; stimulates the liver and
kidneys; rich in minerals to balance the body and
promote healing.

Vitamin and Mineral Content: Rich in calcium,
potassium and sodium. High in vitamin A, C, E and
iron. Moderate amounts of phosphorus, potassium,
manganese, iron, selenium and silicon. Some B-
complex.

Ailments
Age Spots, *Anemia, Blister (external), Blood Pressure
(lowers), Blood Purifier,* Constipation, Corns,
Cramps, Dermatitis, Diabetes, Eczema, *Endurance,*
Fatigue, Fever, *Gallbladder,* Gout, Jaundice,
Hypoglycemia, *Liver Problems,* Metabolism
(stimulates), Psoriasis, Rheumatism, Spleen, Stomach,
Warts.

Devil's Claw
(Harpagophytum procumbens)
Parts Used: Root)

Specific Uses: Liver, stomach, joints and kidneys; used successfully in arthritis, gout and rheumatism; acts as blood cleanser; cleanses vascular walls; good cleanser for the blood and lymph system; natural cleanser to eliminate toxins from the system.

Vitamin and Mineral Content: Rich in iron and magnesium. Moderate amounts of potassium, sodium, selenium, manganese and zinc. Small amounts of phosphorus and silicon.

Ailments
Arteriosclerosis, Arthritis, Bladder (strengthens), *Blood Purifier, Cholesterol, Diabetes,* Gallstones, Gout, *Kidneys (strengthens), Liver Diseases,* Malaria, *Pollution, Rheumatism, Stomach Problems.*

Dong Quai
(Angelica sinensis)
Parts Used: Root

Specific Uses: Uterus, blood, muscles and nerves; useful for all female problems; nourishing to female glands, men use it for migraine headaches; liver problems; heart palpitations; high blood pressure; hypoglycemia and chronic bronchitis; used to dissolve blood clots; nourishes brain; strengthens central nervous system.

Vitamin and Mineral Content: High in vitamin E and iron. Moderate amounts of vitamin A, C, B12, magnesium, phosphorus, potassium and niacin. Small amounts of calcium, sodium, zinc, selenium, manganese, silicon and some B-complex.

Ailments
Abdominal Ache, Aches, *Anemia*, Angina, *Bleeding (internal), Blood Purifier, Brain Nourisher, Breast Abscesses,* Bruises, Chills, Circulation, Clots (blood), Constipation, Cramps, *Female Glands,* Headaches, (migraine) *Hot Flashes,* Hypertension, Hypoglycemia, Lumbago, *Menopause, Menstruation (regulates),* Metabolism, *Nervousness, Pre-menstrual Syndrome,* Preventive, Prolapsed Uterus, Retained Placenta, Stomach, Tonic, Tumors (blood).

Echinacea
(Echinacea angustifolia)
Parts Used: Root

Specific Uses: Blood, Kidneys and lymph glands; blood cleanser; immune system booster; good for teeth abscess, gangrene, pus diseases, swollen lymph glands; effective against bacterial and viral infestations, upper respiratory infections (including tonsillitis and laryngitis), sinus infections; decoction to rinse mouth for pyorrhea and gingivitis.

Vitamin and Mineral Content: High in iron, selenium, zinc, manganese and silicon. Moderate in magnesium, potassium, niacin, vitamin C and E, and some B-complex vitamins. Small amounts of calcium, phosphorus, sodium and vitamin A.

Ailments
Acne, Antiseptic, Bed Sores, Bites (Poisonous), *Blood Builder, Blood Diseases, Blood Poisoning, Blood Purifier, Boils*, Cancer, Carbuncle, Diabetes, Diphtheria, Eczema, Fevers, Gangrene, Glands (swollen), Gonorrhea, Gums, Hemorrhoids, Hydrophobia, Indigestion, *Infections (external), Infections (prevents),* Leg Ulcers, Leukemia, *Lymph Glands,* Mucus, Peritonitis, Pimples, *Prostate,* Pyorrhea, Sores (infected), Spinal Meningitis, Staph Infection, Strep Throat, Syphilis, Tongue and Mouth Infections, Tetanus, Tooth Ache, Typhoid Fever, Tonsillitis, Tuberculosis, Vaccine Infections, Weak Conditions, Wounds.

Eyebright
(Euphrasia officinalis)
Parts Used: The Herb

Specific Uses: Eyes, liver and blood; beneficial to the optic nerves; strengthens eyes, nose and throat; strengthens brain and memory; improves eye health to prevent infections (when used internally and externally); warm oil of eyebright dropped on tooth or in ear relieves infections; compress has helped in bruised black eyes; dissolves styes; eases eye strain.

Vitamin and Mineral Content: Rich in vitamins A, C and silicon. High in calcium, magnesium, manganese, zinc, and niacin, vitamin D and E. Some B-complex, small amounts of sodium, selenium, iodine, copper and zinc.

Ailments
Allergies, Black Eye (compress), *Blood Cleanser,*

Cataracts, Catarrh, Chicken Pox, *Colds,* Congestion, Coughs, Earache, Eye Disorders and Infections, Eye Problems, *Eyes (strengthens),* Gallbladder, Hay Fever, Headaches, Feed Colds, Hoarseness, *Liver Stimulant*, Measles, Memory, Mumps, Sinus Congestion, Spleen, Toothaches, Styes (dissolves).

False Unicorn
(Chamaelirium luteum)
Parts Used: Root

Specific Uses: Uterus and kidneys; beneficial in infertility; nourishes the uterus, ovaries, and male reproductive organs; works with Lobelia to help stop bleeding in miscarriage if fetus is in a healthy condition; good for depression in menopause; heals in leucorrhea; eases vomiting in pregnancy.

Vitamins and Mineral Content: High in calcium, potassium and vitamin C. Moderate amounts of sulphur and traces of zinc.

Ailments
Appetite stimulant, Bright's Disease, *Colic, Coughs,* Depression, Diabetes, *Digestive Problems*, Dropsy, Dyspepsia, Enuresis, Gastro-intestinal Weakness, Headaches, *Kidneys*, Menopause, *Miscarriage (prevents)*, Nausea, Ovaries, *Prostate,* Side Pain, Sterility, *Tape Worm,* Uterine Problems.

Fennel
(Foeniculum vulgare)
Parts Used: Seeds

Specific Uses: Stomach, nerves, intestines and eyes; beneficial for stomach function; relieves cramping; expels gas; dispels phlegm from the throat; removes waste material from the body; fortifies the nerves; purifies the blood.

Vitamin and Mineral Content: High in calcium, magnesium, phosphorus. Moderate in potassium, sulphur, sodium, iron and selenium. Small amounts of zinc, manganese, silicon, vitamins A, C, and E.

Ailments
Appetite Depressant, Bronchitis, *Colic*, Congestion, Convulsions, Coughs, Cramps (abdominal), Digestive Aid, Female Problems, *Gas,* Gout, *Intestinal Problems,* Lactation (promotes), Nervous Disorders, Pin worms, *Sedative for Children,* Spasms.

Fenugreek
(Trigonella foenum-graecum)
Parts Used: Seeds

Specific Uses: Lungs, stomach, intestines and reproductive organs; soothing to the stomach; prevents fatty deposits; soothing for ulcers; kills infections; nourishing for mother's milk; use with lemon juice and honey to reduce fevers; gargle for throat irritations; use seeds boiled in water for nourishment.

Vitamin and Mineral Content: Rich in vitamin A and D--compared to fish liver oils. High in protein, especially lysine and tryptophan, iron. Moderate in calcium, magnesium, phosphorus, potassium, selenium, silicon, and vitamin C. Small amounts of sodium, zinc, manganese, niacin, choline and some B-complex vitamins.

Ailments
Abscess, Allergies, Bad Breath, Blood Poisoning, Boils, Body Odor, *Bronchial Catarrh*, Carbuncles, *Cholesterol (dissolves)*, Fevers (reduce), Inflammations, Lactation, *Lung Infections, Mucus (dissolves), Stomach Irritations*, Throat Gargle, Ulcers, Uterus, Water Retention, Wounds (poultice).

Feverfew
(Chrysanthemum parthenium)
Parts Used: Leaves

Specific Uses: Circulation, nervous system, skin and urinary organs; natural relief for migraine headaches; excellent for relieving colds; inflammation in arthritis; used to help in dizziness, tinnitus and provide circulation to brain and head area (helps in ears, nose and throat).

Vitamin and Mineral Content: Rich in potassium, niacin and other B complex. Moderate amounts of magnesium, selenium, manganese, vitamin B1 and B2, and silicon. Small amounts of vitamin A, C, sodium, iron and zinc.

Ailments
Allergies, Arthritis, Colds, Cramps (menstrual), Dizziness, *Headaches (migraine)*, Hot Flashes, Insect

Bites (external), Menopause Symptoms, Menstruation (sluggish), Nervous Headaches, Nervous Hysteria, Sinus Headaches, Tinnitus.

Garlic
(Allium sativum)
Parts Used: The Bulb

Specific Uses: Respiratory, circulation, digestion, nerves and sinus; dissolves cholesterol and loosens it out of the arteries; kills infections and putrefaction; acts on bacteria, viruses, and internal parasites and worms; reduces blood pressure; builds intestinal flora; purges the system of pollutants; builds the immune system; stimulates the lymphatic system; prevents pneumonia, colds, flu, dysentery, diarrhea and strep infections; kills candida yeast infections.

Vitamin and Mineral Content: High in phosphorus, potassium, sulphur, and zinc. Moderate amounts of selenium, vitamin A and C. Small amounts of calcium, magnesium, sodium, iron, manganese and some B-complex vitamins.

Ailments
Abscess, Anemia, Arthritis, Allergies, *Asthma*, Arteriosclerosis, *Cancer Immunity,* Catarrh, Colds, Diabetes, Diaper Rash, *Digestive Disorders,* Diverticulitis, Dizziness, *Ear Infections,* Emphysema, Fevers, Germ Killer, Heart Disease, *High Blood Pressure*, Hypoglycemia, Infections, *Infectious Disease, Intestinal worms,* Insomnia, Longevity, Low Blood Pressure, Lungs, Lymphatics, Memory, Mucus, Parasites, Regulator of Glands, Scarlet Fever, Skin Problems, Toothache, Toxic Metal Poisoning, Thyroid, Warts, Worms, Yeast Infection.

Gentian
(Gentiana lutea)
Parts Used: The Root

Specific Uses: Stomach, liver, blood, spleen and circulation; helps to balance stomach acid (whether too much or too little); beneficial in cases of exhaustion from chronic disease; weak digestive organs; strengthens the whole body--it warms and enlivens the system.

Vitamin and Mineral Content: High in iron. Contains B-complex, especially inositol and niacin. Contains vitamin F, manganese, silicon, sulphur and zinc.

Ailments
Amenorrhea, Anemia, Antidote for Poisons, *Appetite Stimulant*, Bites (mad dog), Blood, Bruises, Constipation, Cramps, Debility, Diarrhea, *Exhaustion (Physical)*, Female Weakness, Fevers, Gout, Heartburn, Hypoglycemia, *Hysteria, Jaundice*, Joint Inflammation, *Liver Bile*, Mononucleosis, Nausea, Pestilence, Plagues, Scrofula, Spleen Disorders, Stomach Problems, Sprains, *Tonic*, Urinary Infection, Vermin, Vomiting, Worms, Wounds (infected).

Ginger
(Zingiber officinale)
Parts Used: Root

Specific Uses: Stomach, intestines, joints, muscles, used to improve circulation; digestion to promote gastric secretion, stomach cramps; protects to prevent diarrhea, gas, flu, colic, morning sickness, and aids in removal of excess waste from system; ginger and bayberry work together to produce a chemical to protect against viruses.

Vitamin and Mineral Content: High in potassium, manganese and silicon. Moderate amounts of vitamin A, C, B-complex, magnesium and phosphorus. Small amounts of sodium, iron, and zinc.

Ginseng
(Korean Panax schin-seng)
Siberian
(Eleutherococcus)
Wild American
(Panax quinquefolium)
Parts Used: Root

Specific Uses: Circulation, heart and a beneficial effect on the whole body; combats stress and fatigue; increases brain efficiency; preventive and restorative herb; increases physical efficiency; improves concentration span; increases speed and accuracy in work.

Vitamin and Mineral Content: Rich in the B-complex vitamins, and high in selenium. Moderate amounts of A, C, E and G. Small amounts of phosphorus, iron, copper, manganese, cobalt, aluminum, sulphur, silicon, choline, biotin; increases synthesis of nuclear RNA.

Ailments
Age Spots, Anemia, Antidote for some drugs, Appetite, Atherosclerosis, Bleeding (internal), Blood Diseases, *Blood Pressure,* Childbirth (bleeding),

Cholesterol, *Depression,* Digestive Problems, *Endurance (increases),* Euphoria (induces), Fatigue (banishes), Fevers, *Hemorrhage,* Inflammation, Irritability (helps), Liver Diseases, *Longevity,* Lung Problems, Menopause, Menstruation, *Mental vigor,* Nausea, Nervousness, *Physical Vigor,* Radiation Protection, *Sexual Stimulant,* Stress, Ulcers, Vomiting,

Glucomannan
(Amorphophallus konjak)
Parts Used: Root

Specific Uses: Digestion and colon; fiber content to improve gastrointestinal disorders; eliminates harmful bacteria in large intestine; taken before meals produces a fullness to suppress appetite; glucomannan and lecithin can help to prevent heart disease.

Vitamin and Mineral Content: Small amounts of calcium, magnesium, phosphorus, potassium, sodium, iron, selenium, zinc, silicon and manganese. Also vitamin A, C, niacin, B1 and B2.

Ailments
Arteriosclerosis, Cholesterol (serum), *Constipation,* Diabetes, *Diverticula Disease,* Hemorrhoids, *High Blood Pressure*, Hyperglycemia, Hypoglycemia, *Obesity*, Pancreas (reduces stress).

Golden Seal
(Hydrastis canadensis)
Parts Used: Rhizome and Root

Specific Uses: Stomach, intestine, spleen, liver, eyes and mucus membranes; excellent herb when combined with other herbs such as gotu kola for brain food, cascara sagrada as a bowel tonic; use as a gargle for sore throat; mouthwash for pyorrhea and mouth sores; snuffed up nose for nasal catarrh. Use on ringworm, bruises and wounds; stops bleeding.

Vitamin and Mineral Content: High in iron, manganese and silicon. Moderate in magnesium, selenium, zinc, vitamin C and some B-complex vitamins. Small amounts of calcium, phosphorus, potassium, and vitamin A.

Ailments
Antibiotic, Antiseptic, Asthma, Bladder Infection, *Bleeding Internal*, Canker Sores, Cancer, Catarrh, Childhood Disease, Circulation, *Colon Inflammation,* Constipation (chronic), *Diabetes*, Eczema, *Eye Infections,* Hay Fever, Gastritis, Genital Disorders, Gonorrhea, Herpes, *Infection,* Insect Repellent, *Liver Problems*, Lymph Congestion, Mammary and Ovarian Tumors, *Menstruation (excessive),* Morning Sickness, *Mouth Sores,* Ringworm, Rhinitis, Skin Problems, Tonsillitis, Ulceration (skin), Ulcers, Urethritis, *Vaginitis,* Venereal Disease.

Gotu Kola
(Hydrocotyle asiatica)
Parts Used: Their Herb

Specific Uses: Brain, nerves, bladder, kidneys, heart and circulation; strengthens heart, brain and memory; helps balance hormones and relaxes the nerves; rebuilds energy reserve and stamina; combats stress; improves reflexes; "two capsules a day will keep old age away"; blood purifier, useful in schizophrenia, epilepsy and memory loss; neutralizes blood acids.

Vitamin and Mineral Content: High in vitamin A, B-complex, calcium, magnesium, sodium, manganese, silicon and zinc. Moderate in vitamin C, phosphorus, iron and selenium.

Ailments
Blood purifier, Bowel Problems, Depression, *Concentration*, Fatigue, Fevers, Heart (strengthens), *High Blood Pressure*, Infections, Learning Disabilities, Leprosy, Longevity, Memory, Menopause, *Mental Fatigue, Nervous Breakdown, Physical Fatigue,* Rheumatism, Scrofula, *Senility,* Thyroid Stimulant, *Tonic*, Toxins (eliminates), Vitality, Wounds.

Grapevine
(Vitis vinitera)
Parts Used: Leaves and Stems

Specific Uses: Bladder, kidneys, digestive system and tissues; useful to eliminate excess water; strengthens the bladder and kidneys.

Ailments
Diarrhea, *Dropsy*, Dysentery (chronic), Eyes (weak), Gallstones, Kidney Problems, Kidney Stones.

Hawthorn Berries
(Crataegus oxycantha)
Parts Used: Berries

Specific Uses: Heart, circulation, nerves and kidneys; natural food for the heart; prevents hardening of the arteries; heart problems, regulates blood pressure (both high and low); helps in nervous disorders; stressful situations to fortify the nerves and heart.

Vitamin and Mineral Content: High in vitamin C and selenium. Moderate amounts of calcium and potassium. Small amounts of magnesium, phosphorus, and vitamin A. Traces of sodium, iron, manganese, silicon, zinc and some B-complex vitamins.

Ailments
Angina, *Antiseptic, Arteriosclerosis (prevents),* Arthritis, *Cardiac Symptoms,* Congestive heart Failure, Dropsy, *Enlarged Heart, Hardening of the Arteries, Heart Condition, Heart Palpitation, High Blood Pressure, Hypoglycemia,* Insomnia, Kidney

Problems, *Low Blood Pressure,* Miscarriage, Nerves, Rheumatism (inflammatory), Stress, Throat (sore).

Hops
(Humulus lupulus)
Parts Used: Flowers

Specific Uses: Nerves, stomach, blood, liver and gall bladder; relaxing for the nerves; produces restful sleep; strengthens nerves; relaxes tension and relieves anxiety; improves digestion; eases headaches; helps in cramps; intestinal gas; improves liver and gallbladder functions.

Vitamin and Mineral Content: Rich in potassium, niacin, and B-complex vitamins. High amounts of phosphorus and vitamin C. Moderate in calcium, magnesium, selenium, manganese and silicon. Trace amounts of sodium, iron, vitamin A and zinc.

Ailments
Appetite Stimulant, Blood Cleanser, *Bronchitis,* Bruises, Cramps (abdominal), *Delirium, Digestion,* Dizziness, Earache, Female Problems, Fevers (high), Gallstones, *Headaches, Hyperactivity,* Hysteria, *Insomnia*, Itching, Jaundice, Kidney Stones, *Nervousness,* Neuralgia, *Pain, Sexual Desires (excessive),* Skin Irritations, Toothache, Venereal Disease, Water Retention, Whooping Cough, Worms.

Horsetail
(Equisetum arvense)
Parts Used: Whole Herb

Specific Uses: Bones, flesh, cartilage, digestion, kidneys, blood, heart and lungs; contains silicon-- essential in calcium metabolism for hair, nails and teeth; helps in preventing many diseases and maintains internal health; helps bones to heal; builds the immune system and nervous system.

Vitamin and Mineral Content: Rich in silicon and selenium. High in calcium, magnesium, phosphorus, potassium, iron, vitamin C and niacin. Moderate in vitamin A, E, pantothenic acid and PABA. Low amounts of sodium, vitamin B1, B2, chlorine and zinc.

Ailments
Achilles Tendon, Arterial Degeneration, Arteriosclerosis, Arthritis, Atherosclerosis, *Bladder Problems, Bleeding (internal), Bleeding Ulcers, Broken Bones,* Bronchitis, Bursitis, *Circulation Problems, Disc Lesions,* Dropsy, Feet (sweaty), Fevers, *Fractures,* Gallbladder Problems, *Glandular disorders,* Gout, Gums (bleeding), *Hair,* Hemorrhoids, Kidney Disorder, Ligaments, Liver, Lung Problems, Menstruation (excessive), *Nails (brittle), Nervous Tension,* Nose Bleeds, *Osteoporosis,* Paget's Disease, Polyps, Pregnancy and *Skin Problems,* Tonsillitis (gargle), Tuberculosis (Pulmonary), Tumors, *Urinary Ulcers, Urination (suppressed),* Wetting Problems, Wounds.

Ho Shou Wu
(Polygonum multiflorum)
Parts Used: Leaves and Root

Specific Uses: Urinary tract, kidney, bladder and digestive system; relieves backache due to kidney and rheumatic problems; promotes flow of saliva to aid in digestion; prevents gravel deposits; relieves pain when formations pass through the ureters from the kidneys to the bladder; good for inflamed or enlarged prostate gland.

Vitamin and Mineral Content: Moderate in magnesium, phosphorus, iron, selenium, manganese, silicon and sodium. Small amounts of calcium and potassium.

Ailments
Arteriosclerosis, *Arthritis*, Backaches, *Bladder Infections,* Calculi, *Cystitis, Gallstones, Gout, Gonorrhea, Kidney Problems*, Kidney Stones, Pain, Renal Irritations, *Rheumatism, Urinary Problems*

Juniper
(Juniperis communis)
Parts Used: Berries

Specific Uses: Kidneys and stomach; good to clean the stomach of putrefaction; antiseptic in cystitis; strong diuretic (use in small doses); relieves catarrh of bladder; leucorrhea and gonorrhea.

Vitamin and Mineral Content: High in vitamin C. Moderate amounts of calcium, potassium, manganese and silicon. Small amounts of magnesium, iron, vitamin A, niacin and sulphur. Trace amounts of phosphorus, sodium, selenium, zinc and vitamin B-complex.

Ailments
Ague, *Bleeding*, Bladder Problems, Catarrhal Inflammations, *Colds,* Colic, Coughs, Convulsions, Cramps, Cystitis, Diabetes, *Dropsy*, Gas, Gonorrhea, Gums (bleeding), *Infections,* Insect Bites (poisonous), *Kidney Infections,* Leucorrhea, Menstruation (regulates), *Pancreas,* Piles, Snakebites, Sores, Tuberculosis, Typhoid Fever, *Uric Acid (build up),* *Urinary disorders, Water Retention,* Worms.

Kelp
(Fucus vesiculosis)
Parts Used: Whole Plant

Specific Uses: Thyroid, nerves, brain, kidneys, and bladder; eliminates waste and toxic metals; regulates metabolism; helps glands to function properly, very nourishing; detoxifies intestines to relieve nervous disorders; prevents falling hair; strengthens tissues in the brain and heart.

Vitamin and Mineral Content: Contains approximately thirty trace and major minerals. Rich in iodine, calcium, magnesium, potassium, sodium, sulphur, silicon and iron. High in some B-complex vitamins. Moderate amounts of phosphorus, selenium, manganese and zinc. Small amounts of vitamin A, C, E and G. Contains anti-sterility vitamin S, as well as vitamin K.

Ailments
Adrenal Glands, Arteries (cleans), Asthma, *Birth Defects (Preventive), Colitis, Complexion*, Constipation, Diabetes, Digestion, *Eczema, Fingernails,* Gallbladder, Gas, Goiter, Hair Loss, Headaches, *High Blood Pressure,* Kidneys, Lead Poisoning, Liver, Morning Sickness, Nervous disorder, Neuritis, Obesity, Pancreas, *Pituitary Glands. Pregnancy,* Prostate (tones), *Radiation,* Skin, *Thyroid Gland*, Tumors, Uterus (weak), Vitality (low), Water Retention, Worms, Wrinkles.

Lady's Slipper
(Cypripedium pubescens)
Parts Used: Root

Specific Uses: Nerves; relives muscular pain; excellent for chronic brain syndrome such as stroke good for hysteria, nervous headaches, irritability and most nervous disorders; rebuilds damaged and frayed nerve sheath; quick relief for nervous disorders with no side effects.

Vitamin and Mineral Content: High in calcium, selenium and zinc. Moderate amounts of magnesium, phosphorus, potassium, manganese, iron and silicon. Small amounts of B-complex and sodium.

Ailments
Abdominal Pain, After Pains (birth), *Chorea,* Colic, Cramps, Cystic Fibrosis, Epilepsy, Headaches, (nervous), *Hysteria, Insomnia,* Muscle Spasms, *Nervousness,* Neuralgia, *Pain, Restlessness,* Tremors, Typhoid Fever.

Licorice
(Glycyrrhiza glabra)
Parts Used: Root

Specific Uses: Lungs, stomach, intestine, spleen and liver; has general effect on the whole system; stimulates estrogen and cortisone production when needed in the body; nourishes the adrenals; helps the body to cope with stress and worry; helps in controlling arterial health.

Vitamin and Mineral Content: Rich in magnesium and sodium. High amounts of iron, potassium and silicon. Moderate amounts of calcium, manganese, vitamin C, niacin and B-complex vitamins. Small amounts of vitamin E, B2, pantothenic acid, biotin, and zinc. Trace amounts of selenium, vitamin A and lecithin.

Ailments
Adrenal Exhaustion, *Addison's Disease*, Age Spots, Arteriosclerosis, Arthritis, *Blood Cleanser*, Bronchial Congestion, Circulation, *Colds,* Constipation, Coughs, Cushing's Disease, Dropsy, *Drug Withdrawal,* Emphysema, Endurance, *Energy, Female Complaints,* Fevers, Flu, Heart (strengthens), *Hoarseness, Hypoglycemia*, Impotency, Liver, *Lung Problems*, Parkinson's Disease, *Phlegm (expels), Throat (sore), Tonic,* Ulcers, Vitality.

Lobelia
(Lobelia inflata)
Parts Used: The Herb

Specific Uses: Nerves, lungs, stomach, muscles, circulation and a beneficial effect on the whole body; valuable in dry, barking or hacking coughs--helps to loosen hardened mucus (small doses work best); good for spasmodic lung and respiratory conditions; powerful relaxant in many diseases; relieves cramps, spasms, and lock-jaw; use on gums of teething babies; balances the glands for proper function; valuable in distress crisis.

Vitamin and Mineral Content: High in vitamin C. Moderate amounts of manganese, iron, potassium, sulphur, vitamin A and B1. Small amounts of calcium, magnesium, phosphorus, sodium and selenium. Trace amounts of B12 and zinc.

Ailments
Allergies, *Arthritis (tincture)*, *Asthma*, Blood Poisoning, *Bronchitis, Catarrh*, Childhood Diseases, Circulation, *Colds,* Colic, *Congestion,* Constipation, *Convulsions, Cough,* Cramps, *Croup (tincture), Earache (tincture), Ear Infections,* Eczema, *Epilepsy*, Female Problems, *Fevers. Food Poisoning*, Headache, Heart, Hepatitis, Hydrophobia, *Lock Jaw (tincture), Lung Problems, Miscarriage, Nervousness, Pain,* Palsy, Pleurisy, *Pneumonia,* Poison Ivy and Oak, Rheumatism, Rabies, Ringworm (tincture), Scarlet Fever, Shock, *Spasms,* Syphilis, Teeth, Tetanus, Tonsillitis, Toothaches, Vomiting (small doses), *Whooping Cough, Worms,* Wounds.

Marshmallow
(Althea officinalis)
Parts Used: Root

Specific Uses: Intestines, kidney's and bladder; soothing for lung problems; healing to kidneys; good for diarrhea, dysentery and ulcers; heals in inflammatory conditions of the digestive tract; used in bronchitis, respiratory catarrh and coughs; used externally on varicose veins, abscesses and boils.

Vitamin and Mineral Content: High in vitamin A, magnesium, iron and selenium. Rich in protein and calcium. Moderate amounts of vitamin C, phosphorus, potassium and manganese. Small amounts of niacin, B1, B2, silicon and zinc.

Mullein
(Verbascum thapsus)
Parts Used: Leaves

Specific Uses: Lungs, glands, and lymph; good for bronchitis and lung congestion; useful for hard cough with soreness; soothes inflammations of the throat and digestive system; swollen lymph glands; sinus congestions, tumors and whooping cough.

Vitamin and Mineral Content: Rich in iron. High in calcium, magnesium, manganese and sulphur. Moderate amounts of vitamin A, C, D and B complex. Also contains moderate amounts of potassium, sodium and silicon. Small amounts of phosphorus, selenium and zinc.

Ailments
Asthma, Bleeding (bowel and lungs), Bowel Complaints, *Bronchitis,* Bruises, Colds, *Coughs,* Cramps, *Croup, Diaper Rash,* Diarrhea, Dropsy, *Dysentery, Earaches (oil),* Female Problems, Gas, Glands (cleans), Hay Fever, Hemorrhage, Hemorrhoids, Hoarseness, *Insomnia, Lymphatic System,* Lung Problems, *Nervousness, Pain (relieves), Pleurisy,* Pneumonia, *Sinus Congestion,* Sores, *Tuberculosis,* Venereal Diseases, Wounds.

Oatstraw
(Avena sativa)
Parts Used: Stems

Specific Uses: Nerves, uterus, stomach and lungs; calming for the nerves; relaxes aches and pains and relieves body tension; nutritious tonic for weak nerves; builds immune system; good for digestion, gastroenteritis, dyspepsia and ulcers; beneficial for ovarian and uterine disorders; gives the body a feeling of well-being; loosens mucus in lungs and expels it; stores silicon (needed in the skin and hair).

Vitamin and Mineral Content: Rich in calcium and magnesium. High in silicon and phosphorus. Moderate amounts of vitamin A, B1, B2, and E, sodium, iron and selenium. Small amounts of potassium, manganese and zinc.

Ailments
Arthritis, *Bed Wetting*, Bladder, Boils, Bones (brittle), Bursitis, Constipation, Eyes, Gallbladder, Gout, *Indigestion, Insomnia, Heart (strengthens)*, Kidneys, Liver, Lungs, *Nerves*, Pancreas, Paralysis, Rheumatism, *Urinary Organs*, Wounds.

Oregon Grape
(Berberis aquifolium)
Parts Used: Rhizome and Root

Specific Uses: Liver, blood, stomach, intestines, and skin; excellent blood purifier; beneficial to clear chronic diseases such as acne, eczema, psoriasis, herpes and syphilis; helps all diseases due to impure blood.

Vitamin and Mineral Content: Contains vitamin C, D and E. Also manganese, silicon, sodium and zinc.

Ailments
Acne, Appetite (increases), Arthritis (rheumatoid), *Blood Purifier,* Bowels, Bronchitis, Constipation

(chronic), *Digestion (promotes)*, Eczema, Hepatitis, Herpes, *Jaundice*, Kidneys, Leucorrhea, *Liver*, Lymph Glands, Malaria, *Psoriasis*, Rheumatism, Rocky Mountain Spotted Fever, Scarlet Fever, Scrofula, *Skin Diseases, Staph Infection*, Strength (increases), Syphilis, Typhoid Fever, Uterine Disease, Vaginitis (Douche).

Parsley
(Carum petroselinum)
Parts Used: Leaves

Specific Uses: Kidneys, bladder, stomach, liver and gallbladder; nourishing for the stomach--helps in indigestion and assimilation; tones the blood vessels, arteries and capillaries; stimulates the immune system; helps in obstructions of the kidneys, liver and spleen.

Vitamin and Mineral Content: Rich in vitamin A, C, iron, chlorophyll, potassium and sodium. High in calcium, phosphorus, sulphur and B-complex. Small amounts of selenium, silicon, zinc and other trace minerals.

Ailments
Allergies, Arthritis, Asthma, *Bladder Infection, Blood Builder, Blood Cleanser*, Blood Pressure (low), Breath (bad), Cancer, Coughs, Digestion, *Dropsy*, Eyes, *Gallstones*, Gonorrhea, Gout, Hay Fever, *Jaundice, Kidney Inflammation*, Liver, Lumbago, Menstruation (promotes), Pituitary, Prostate, Rheumatism, Sciatica, Thyroid, Tumors, *Urine Retention*, Varicose Veins, Venereal Diseases.

Passion Flower
(Passiflora incarnata)
Parts Used: The Herb

Specific Uses: Nerves and circulation; produces refreshing sleep for emotionally upset, mentally worried and when overtired; relaxes coughs; good for hysteria, muscle twitching and irritability; good to strengthen the nervous system; used in tension illnesses--especially asthma.

Vitamin and Mineral Content: High in calcium. Moderate in vitamin A and C.,

Ailments
Asthma (spasmodic), Convulsions, Cough (nervous), Diarrhea, Dysentery. Epilepsy, *Eye Infection*, Eye Strain, *Eye Tensions, Fevers,* Headaches, High Blood Pressure, Hysteria, Insomnia, *Menopause*, Menstruation (painful), Muscle Spasms, Nervous Breakdown, Neuralgia, Pain, Vision (dimness).

Pau D'Arco
(Tabebuia avellanedae)
Parts Used: Inner Bark

Specific Uses: Blood, digestive, circulation, beneficial effect on the whole body; kills viruses; very effective against cancers (all kinds); increases resistance to diseases; builds immune system; helps insomnia and anxiety state; heals wounds and the combats infections.

Vitamin and Mineral Content: Rich in calcium and iron. Moderate in selenium. Small amounts of magnesium, manganese, vitamin C and zinc. Trace amounts of phosphorus, potassium, sodium, vitamin A and some B-complex.

Ailments
Anemia, Arteriosclerosis, Arthritis, Asthma, *Blood Builder,* Bronchitis, *Cancer (all types),* Colitis, Cystitis, Diabetes, Eczema, Eyelids (paralysis), Fistulas, Gastritis, Gonorrhea, Hemorrhages, Hernias, Hodgkins Disease, Infections, *Leukemia*, Liver Ailments, Lupus, Nephritis, Osteomyelitis, *Pain (Relieves),* Parkinson's Disease, Polyps, Prostatitis, Psoriasis, Pyorrhea, Rheumatism, Ringworm, *Skin Cancer*, Skin Sores, Spleen Infections, Syphilis, *Tonic*, Ulcers, Varicose Ulcers, Varicose Veins, Venereal Disease, Wounds.

Papaya
(Carica papaya)
Parts Used: Fruit

Specific Uses: Digestive system, colon and blood; protein assimilation; relieves stomach disorders; soothing for the intestinal tract and diarrhea.

Vitamin and Mineral Content: Rich in vitamin A, magnesium and sodium. High in vitamin C, B-complex with PABA and pantothenic acid. Moderate amounts of vitamins D, E, G, K, and zinc. Small amounts of phosphorus, potassium, iron, manganese and niacin. Trace amounts of calcium and sulphur.

Ailments
Allergies, Blood Clotting, *Colon*, Burns, Constipation, *Digestion,* Diarrhea (chronic), Freckles

(juice), *Gas*, Hemorrhage, *Insect Bites, Intestinal Tract,* Sores, Stomach Problems, Worms, Wounds.

Peach Bark
(Prunus persica)
Parts Used: Bark and Leaves

Specific Uses: Stomach, liver, bladder, bowels and nerves; aids digestive tract; excellent for bladder problems; morning sickness; useful for bronchitis and lung congestion.

Vitamin and Mineral Content: High in magnesium, phosphorus and potassium. Moderate amounts of iron and selenium. Small amounts of calcium and manganese, sodium, silicon and zinc.

Ailments
Bladder, Bronchitis (chronic), Congestion (chest), Constipation, Gastritis, Insomnia, Jaundice, Morning Sickness, Mucus, *Nausea*, Nervousness, Sores, Stomach Problems, Uterine Problems *Water Retention*, Whooping Cough, *Worms,* Wounds.

Peppermint
(Mentha piperita)
Parts Used: Leaves

Specific Uses: Stomach, intestines, muscles and circulation; excellent to use in nausea, vomiting, chills, colic, fevers, gas and diarrhea; natural remedy for digestive problems; cleansing for body; soothing for relaxation.

Vitamin and Mineral Content: Rich in vitamin A

and B-complex. High in calcium, magnesium, phosphorus, potassium, sodium and iron. Moderate amounts of selenium and manganese. Small amounts of vitamin C, silicon and zinc.

Ailments
Appetite, Bowel Spasms, Chills, Cholera, *Colds, Colic,* Constipation, Convulsions, Cramps (stomach), Depression (mental), *Digestions,* Dizziness, Fainting, *Fever,* Flu, *Gas, Headaches,* Heart, *Heartburn,* Hysteria, Insomnia, Measles, Menstruation Pain, Morning sickness, Mouthwash, Nausea, Nerves, Neuralgia, Nightmares, Seasickness, *Shock,* Stomach Spasms, Vomiting.

Psyllium
(Plantago ovata)
Parts Used: Seeds

Specific Uses: Bowels and intestines; excellent cleanser for colitis, hemorrhoids, and ulcers; eliminates toxins in colon; rebuilds colon; creates bulk and fiber lacking in typical American diet.

Vitamin and Mineral Content: High in zinc. Moderate amounts of Vitamin A, C, potassium and selenium. Small amounts of calcium, sodium, iron and manganese. Trace amounts of magnesium, phosphorus, silicon and some B-complex vitamins.

Ailments
Colitis, *Colon Blockage, Constipation, Diverticulitis,* Dysentery, Gonorrhea, Hemorrhoids, Intestinal Tract, Ulcers, Urinary Tract.

Red Clover
(Trifolium pratense)
Parts Used: Flowers

Specific Uses: Blood, liver, lymph, nerves, lungs and digestion; useful for cancer because of its beneficial effect on protein assimilation; wonderful blood cleanser and tonic.

Vitamin and Mineral Content: High in calcium, magnesium, potassium, vitamin C, iron and niacin. Moderate amounts of manganese, phosphorus and some B-complex vitamins. Small amounts of vitamin A, B2, selenium, sodium, silicon and zinc.

Ailments
Acne, Appetite, Arthritis, Athlete's Foot, *Blood Purifier,* Boils, *Bronchitis,* Burns, *Cancer,* Childhood Disease, Constipation, Coughs, Digestive Problems, Douche, Eczema, Eyewash, Flu, Hay Fever, Leprosy, Leukemia, Liver, *Nervous Energy,* Psoriasis, Rheumatism, Rickets, Scarlet Fever, Scrofula, Skin Cancer, Skin Diseases, Sores, *Spasmodic Affections,* Stomach Cancer, Syphilis, *Toxins*, Ulcers, Urinary Problems, Vitality and Weak Chest, Wheezing, Whooping Cough, Wounds (fresh).

Red Raspberry
(Rubus idaeus)
Parts Used: Leaves

Specific Uses: Stomach, liver, blood, genitourinary and muscles; strengthens uterus walls and the female reproductive system; excellent female tonic; soothing to the mucus membranes and kidneys.

Vitamin and Mineral Content: Rich in manganese, iron and niacin. High in calcium, magnesium, selenium, vitamin A and C. Moderate amounts of phosphorus, potassium and B-complex vitamins. Trace amounts of sodium, silicon, and zinc.

Ailments
Afterpains, Bowel Problems, Bronchitis, Canker Sores, *Childbirth,* Cholera, Colds, Constipation, Diabetes, *Diarrhea,* Digestion, Dysentery, Eye Wash, *Female organs, Fevers, Flu,* Hemorrhoids, Labor Pains, Lactation, Leucorrhea, Measles, Menstruation, *Morning Sickness, Mouth Sores, Nausea,* Nervousness, *Pregnancy,* Stomach, Teething, Throat (sore), Thrush, Ulcers, Urinary Problems, Uterus (prolapsed), *Vomiting,* Wounds.

Rose Hips
(Rosa species)
Parts Used: Fruit (hips)

Specific Uses: Blood, nerves and heart; good all-around tonic for most conditions; excellent for nervous and stressful situations.

Vitamin and Mineral Content: Rich in vitamin A, C, E, rutin and sodium. High in amounts of calcium, iron, selenium, manganese and B-complex. Moderate amounts of calcium. Small amounts of magnesium, potassium, manganese, sulphur and silicon. Trace amounts of vitamin D, P and zinc.

Ailments
Arteriosclerosis, Bites, *Blood Purifier,* Bruises, *Cancer,* Circulation, *Colds,* Contagious Diseases,

Cramps, Dizziness, Earaches, Fever, *Flu*, Headaches, *Infections*, Kidney Stones, Mouth Sores, *Nervousness*, Psoriasis, Stings, Stress, *Throat (sore).*

Safflower
(Carthamus tinctorius)
Parts Used: Flowers

Specific Uses: Skin, stomach, kidneys, pancreas and nerves; useful to aid in digestion; helps digest oils good to eliminate cholesterol and uric acid.

Vitamin and Mineral Content: High in potassium and sodium. Moderate amounts of magnesium, phosphorus, iron, selenium and vitamin K. Small amounts of calcium, manganese, silicon and zinc.

Ailments
Arthritis, Boils (external), Bronchitis, Chickenpox, Colitis, *Delirium, Digestion, Fevers,* Gallbladder, Gas, Gout, *Jaundice*, Heartburn, Heart (strengthens), Hypoglycemia, Hysteria, *Liver,* Measles, Menstruation, Mumps, Pancreas, *Phlegm*, Poison Ivy, Scarlet Fever, *Sweating*, Tuberculosis, *Uric Acid, Urinary Problems.*

Saffron
(Crocus sativus)
Parts Used: Flowers

Specific Uses: Digestion, colon, skin and blood; can be used the same as safflower; helps in digestion of oils; helpful in uric acid build-up.

Vitamin and Mineral Content: Contains moderate

amounts of vitamin, B2, potassium, calcium, phosphorus and sodium.

Ailments

Arthritis, Bronchitis, Coughs, Digestion, *Fevers,* Gas, *Gout,* Headaches, Heartburn, Hyperglycemia, Hypoglycemia, Insomnia, Jaundice, *Measles*, Menstruation, Psoriasis, *Rheumatism, Scarlet Fever*, Skin Diseases, Stomach Disorders, Tuberculosis, Ulcers (internal), Uterine Hemorrhages, Water Retention.

Sage
(Salvia officinalis)
Parts Used: Leaves

Specific Uses: Bowels, sinuses, bladder, mucus, membranes and nerves; good for head and brain; memory; gargle for sore throat; inflamed gums; poultice for ulcers; sores and skin eruptions.

Vitamin and Mineral Content: High in calcium, potassium, B1 and zinc. Moderate amounts of magnesium, sodium, iron, vitamin A, niacin, B2 and B-complex vitamins. Small amounts of phosphorus, manganese, silicon, sulphur, silicon, sodium and vitamin C. Trace amounts of selenium.

Ailments

Brain (stimulates), Bladder Infection, Blood Infections, Colds, *Coughs*, Diarrhea, *Digestion*, Dysentery, *Fevers,* Flu, Gravel, *Gums (sore),* Hair Growth, Headaches, Lactation (stops), Laryngitis, Lung Congestion, *Memory (improves), Mouth Sores, Nausea, Nerves*, Night Sweats, Palsy, Parasites,

Phlegm, Sinus Congestion, Snake Bites, Teeth Cleanser, *Throat (sore),* Tonsillitis, Ulcers, Worms, Yeast Infection.

Sarsaparilla
(Smilax ornata)
Parts Used: Root

Specific Uses: Blood, skin, circulation and intestines; balances female hormones; stimulates the body's defense system.

Vitamin and Mineral Content: High amount of iron. Moderate amounts of potassium, manganese, silicon, sodium and B-complex. Small amounts of calcium, magnesium, phosphorus, sulphur, copper, iodine and zinc. Also small amounts of vitamins A, C and D.

Ailments
Age Spots, *Blood Purifier*, Catarrh, Colds, Dropsy, Eyes (sore), Fevers, *Gas,* Gout, *Joint Aches, Hormone Herb,* Menopause, Physical Debility, Psoriasis, Rheumatism, (chronic), Ringworm, Sexual Impotence, Scrofula, Skin diseases, Skin Parasites, Sores, Tetters, Venereal Diseases.

Saw Palmetto
(Serenoa serrulata)
Parts Used: Fruit

Specific Uses: Lungs, throat, reproductive organs and kidneys; Strengthens glandular tissues; good for wasting diseases.

Vitamin and Mineral Content: Contains some vitamin A.

Ailments
Asthma, Bladder Disease, *Breasts*, Bronchitis (chronic), Catarrhal Problems, Colds (head), Diabetes, *Digestion,* Frigidity, *Glands*, Gonorrhea, Hot Flashes, Impotence, Kidney Diseases, Lung Congestion, Mucus Discharges, Nerves, Neuralgia, Prostate (enlarged), *Reproductive Organs, Sex Stimulant*, Sterility,Tonic, Urinary Problems, *Weight (Increases)*.

Scullcap
(Scutellaria lateriflora)
Parts Used: The Herb

Specific Uses: Nerves and stomach; special influence on the spinal cord and nervous system; good for digestive problems, circulation, emotional conflict, worry and restlessness.

Vitamin and Mineral Content: Rich in zinc. High in calcium, magnesium and potassium. Moderate in manganese, silicon, vitamin A, B1, C and E. Small amounts of phosphorus, iron, selenium, niacin and vitamin B2. Trace amounts of sodium.

Ailments
Aches, Alcoholism, Blood Pressure, Childhood Diseases, *Convulsions*, Delirium, Drug Withdrawal, *Epilepsy, Fevers (reduces)*, Fits, Hangover, Headaches, *High Blood Pressure*, Hydrophobia, Hypertension, Hysteria, Hypoglycemia, *Infertility*, Insanity, *Insomnia*, Lock-haw, *Nerves*, Nervous Tension, Neuralgia, Pain, Palsy, Parkinson's Disease,

Poisonous bites, Pre-menstrual Tension, Rabies, *Restlessness*, Rheumatism, Rickets, Spasms, Spinal Meningitis, Stress, St. Virus Dance, Thyroid Problems, Tremors, Urinary.

Slippery Elm
(Ulmus fulva)
Parts Used: Inner Bark

Specific Uses: Beneficial effect on the whole body; strengthens, heals and soothes inflamed or irritated areas; absorbs noxious gases; neutralizes stomach acidity; equal to oatmeal in vitamin and mineral content.

Vitamin and Mineral Content: High in protein and B-complex vitamins. Moderate amounts of vitamin A and selenium. Small amounts of vitamin E, F, K, P and magnesium. Trace amounts of iron, phosphorus, potassium, silicon, sodium, and zinc.

Ailments
Appendicitis, *Asthma*, Bladder Problems, Boils, Bowels, *Bronchitis, Burns,* Cancer, *Colitis, Colon, Coughs,* Constipation, Croup, *Diaper Rash, Diarrhea, Digestion*, Diphtheria, Dysentery, Female Problems, Hemorrhoids, Herpes, Inflammations, Laxative, *Lung Problems,* Pain, Phlegm, Pneumonia, Poison Ivy (external); Sores, *Syphilis*, Throat (sore), Tuberculosis, Tumors, Ulcers, Urinary Problems, Vaginal Irritations, Worms, Wounds, Whooping Cough.

Stevia
(Stevia rebaudiana)
Parts Used: Leaves

Specific Uses: Sweetener and flavoring agent. Two drops equals one teaspoonful of white sugar. Three hundred times sweeter than sucrose (white sugar).

Vitamin and Mineral Content: High in magnesium, phosphorus, potassium and selenium. Moderate in manganese, silicon and sodium. Small amounts of calcium, iron and zinc.

Ailments
Alcoholism, Candida, Diabetes, *Energy, Hypoglycemia, Pre-menstrual Syndrome*, Smoking (withdrawal), Stress.

Spirulina
(Food Plankton, Blue-green algae)

Specific Uses: Beneficial for all parts of the body; contains all eight essential amino acids in the correct proportion; contain enzymes to help release nutrients for nourishment; rich in chlorophyll satisfies the body's need for proper nutrients.

Vitamin and Mineral Content: Rich in protein, and contains all the B-complex vitamins, vitamin A and E. Rich in chelated minerals, potassium, magnesium, selenium, zinc, iron, phosphorus, calcium and manganese.

Ailments
Anemia, Diabetes, Digestion, *Energy*, Hepatitis, *Obesity,* Pancreatitis, *Stamina, Stress, Survival Food,* Ulcers, Vitamin Source.

Uva Ursi
(Arctostaphylos uva-ursi) **(Bearberry)**
Parts Used: Leaves

Specific Uses: Kidneys and urinary tract; healing and soothing to the genito-urinary organs; capable of dissolving kidney stones; strengthens the spleen.

Vitamin and Mineral Content: High in vitamin A, iron and manganese. Moderate amounts of calcium, selenium and silicon. Small amounts of vitamin C, niacin, magnesium and potassium. Trace amounts of B-complex vitamins, phosphorus, sodium and zinc.

Ailments
Arthritis, Bedwetting, *Bladder Infections,* Bronchitis, *Bright's Disease, Cystitis, Diabetes,* Diarrhea, Dysentery, Female Troubles, Gallstones, *Gonorrhea,* Gravel, Hemorrhoids, *Kidney Infections,* Liver, Lung Congestion, Menstruation (excessive), *Nephritis,* Pancreas, Prostate Weakness, *Spleen,* Uric Acid (excess), *Urethritis (chronic), Uterine, Ulceration.*

Valerian
(Valeriana officinalis)
Parts Used: Root

Specific Uses: Nerves; nourishing and soothing to the nervous system; helps reduce anxiety, tension, and hysteria.

Vitamin and Mineral Content: Rich in calcium, magnesium and potassium. High amounts of manganese, niacin and selenium. Moderate amounts of iron, B-complex vitamins and choline. Trace amounts of phosphorus, sodium, silicon, and zinc. Traces of vitamin A and C.

Ailments
Alcoholism, Bronchial Spasm, Colds, Coughs, *Convulsions,* Despondency, Drug Addiction, Epilespy, Gravel in Bladder, Head Congestion, *High Blood Pressure, Hysteria, Hypochondria*, Insomnia, Measles, Menstruation (promotes), Migraine Headaches, Muscle Pain, *Nervousness, Pain,* Palpitation, Palsy, Scarlet Fever, Shock, Spasm, Stress, Tension, Ulcers, Worms (expels).

White Oak
(Quercus alba)
Parts Used: Bark

Specific Uses: Skin, gastro-intestinal tract, kidneys; contains properties for clotting, shrinking and disinfecting; used on sores and wounds to prevent infections; healing for herpes, thrush, varicose veins and yeast infections.

Vitamin and Mineral Content: Rich in calcium with high amounts of manganese. Moderate amounts of iodine, iron, selenium, and sulphur. Small amounts of vitamin A, C, niacin, B1, B2, B12, magnesium, phosphorus, potassium, silicon, sodium and zinc.

Ailments
Bites (insect and snake), Bladder Problems, *Bleeding (internal and external), Bloody Urine*, Cancer (prostate), Dental Problems, Diarrhea, Fever (reduces), Gangrene, Glandular Swellings, Goiter, Gums (sore), *Hemorrhoids*, Herpes, Indigestion, Kidneys, Liver, *Menstrual Problems, Mouth Sores,* Nausea, Pyorrhea, *Skin Irritations,* Spleen Problems, *Teeth, Throat (strep)*, Thrush, Tonsillits, *Ulcers*, Uterus, Vagina, *Varicose Veins,* Venereal Diseases, Vomiting, *Worms (pin)*, Wounds (external), Yeast Infections.

White Willow
(Salix alba)
Parts Used: Bark

Specific Uses: Nerves, stomach, kidneys, bowels, intestines and head area; used for pain and fever instead of aspirin, useful for chronic diarrhea in children; useful for flu and colds.

Vitamin and Mineral Content: High amounts of calcium, magnesium, phosphorus and zinc. Moderate amounts of manganese, potassium and selenium. Small amounts of B-complex vitamins, iron and silicon. Trace amounts of vitamin A, C and sodium.

Ailments
Arthritis, Bleeding (internal), Bursitis, Chills, Corns, Dandruff, Diarrhea, Dysentery, Earache, *Eczema, Fever,* Flu, Gout, Hay Fever, *Headache,* Heartburn, Infection, Inflammation, Lumbago, Muscle (sore), *Nervousness,* Neuralgia, Night Sweats, Ovarian Pain, *Pain, Rheumatism,* Sex Depressant, Tonsillitis, *Ulceration,* Worms, *Wounds.*

Wild Yam
(Dioscorea villosa)
Parts Used: Root

Specific Uses: Muscles, joints; uterus, liver and gall bladder; good for female problems; abdominal cramps and bowels spasms; relaxes the muscular fibers; soothes the nerves and relieves pain; valued in nervousness, restlessness and nausea.

Vitamin and Mineral Content: High amounts of zinc, moderate in vitamin A, B-complex, iron and manganese. Small amounts of vitamin C, calcium, magnesium, phosphorus, potassium and selenium. Trace amounts of niacin, silicon and sodium.

Ailments
Addison's Disease, *Arthritis, Asthma (spasmodic), Birth Control, Boils, Bowel Spasms,* Bronchitis, Catarrh (stomach), Cholera, *Colic (bilious)),* Cushing's Disease, *Gas,* Glandular Balance, Hiccough (spasmodic), Hypoglycemia, Hyperglycemia, Jaundice, *Liver Problems Menstrual Cramps, Muscle Pain,* Miscarriage (prevents), *Nausea (pregnancy),* Nervousness, Neuralgia, Rheumatism, Scabies, Spasms, Whooping Cough.

Wood Betony
(Betonica officinalis)
Parts Used: The Herb

Specific Uses: Nerves and liver; excellent for spleen disorders; valuable as a natural stimulant; acts as a mild sedative to the central nervous system; good for the immune system; protects against epidemic diseases.

Vitamin and Mineral Content: Rich in calcium with moderate amounts of magnesium, manganese, phosphorus and potassium.

Ailments
Asthma (bronchial), Bladder, Bleeding (internal), Blood (improves), Bronchitis, Bruises, Convulsions, *Delirium*, Diarrhea, Epilespy, Fainting, *Fevers,* Gout, *Headaches (migraine)*, Heartburn, Heart Stimulant, *Hysteria,* Indigestion, Insanity, *Jaundice*, Kidney, *Liver Problems,* Lung Congestion, *Nervousness,* Neuralgia, Night Sweats, Pain, Palsy, Parasites, Perspiration, Sprains, Stomach Cramps, Varicose Veins, Ulcers, *Worms*.

Yarrow
(Achillea millefolium)
Parts Used: Flower

Specific Uses: Circulation and beneficial to all parts of the body; stops bleeding (internal and external); good for childhood diseases with skin eruptions; excellent preventive herb.

Vitamin and Mineral Content: High in potassium

and phosphorus with moderate amounts of B-complex (especially choline and inositol), magnesium, manganese, selenium and silicon. Small amounts of vitamin A, C, E, F (fatty acids) and P (bioflavonoids). Trace amounts of K, iron, sodium and zinc.

Ailments
Abrasion, Malaria, Appetite (stimulates), Bladder, *Blood Cleanser, Bowels (hemorrhage),* Bright's Disease, Bronchitis, Bruises, Burns, Cancer, *Catarrh, Chicken Pox. Colds,* Cramps, Cuts, Diarrhea (infant), Epilepsy, *Fevers, Flu,* Hair (falling out), Headaches, Hysteria, Jaundice, *Lungs (hemorrhage),* Malaria, *Measles*, Menstrual Bleeding, Nipples (sore), *Nose Bleeds,* Piles, *Perspiration (obstructed),* Pleurisy, Pneumonia, Rheumatism, Smallpox, Stomach Problems, Sweating (promotes), Throat (inflamed), Typhoid Fever, Ulcers, Urine Retention.

Yellow Dock
(Rumex crispus)
Parts Used: Root

Specific Uses: Blood, skin, spleen, liver and gall bladder; balances body chemistry with its high mineral content; nourishes the glands; builds up the immune system.

Vitamin and Mineral Content: Rich in vitamin A, C, iron and manganese. High in b-complex vitamins, magnesium, phosphorus and selenium. Contains moderate amounts of calcium, potassium and niacin. Trace amounts of sodium and silicon.

Ailments
Anemia, Arsenic Poisoning, Bladder, Blood Disorders, Blood Purifier, Bowels (bleeding), Bronchitis (chronic), Cancer, Constipation, Dyspepsia, Ears (running), Itching, Eyelids (ulcerated), Female Weakness, jaundice, Leprosy, Leukemia, Liver, Congestion, Lungs (bleeding), Lymphatic Problems, Rheumatism, Scurvy, Skin Problems, Spleen, Stomach Problems, Thyroid Glands, Tumors, Ulcers.

Yerba Santa
(Eridictyon californicum)
Parts Used: Leaves

Specific Uses: Lungs and stomach; used for all kinds of bronchial congestion; improves digestion; good for allergies and hay fever.

Ailments
Allergies, *Asthma,* Bladder, Catarrh, *Bronchial Congestion,* Catarrh, *Colds,* Coughs (dry), Diarrhea, Dysentery, Fever, Flu, Headaches, Hemorrhoids, *Hay Fever*, Kidney Problems, Laryngitis (chronic), Rheumatism, Sinus Drainage, Stomach Aches, Throat (sore), Vomiting.

Yucca
(Yucca glauca)
Parts Used: Root

Specific Uses: Blood, digestion; beneficial for all parts of the body; contains steroid saponins which are found to be an anti-stress agent; reduces toxins in the alimentary canal, which relieves associated problems such as asthma, arthritis and migraine headaches.

Vitamin and Mineral Content: Contains moderate amounts of calcium, sodium, zinc and B-complex vitamins. Small amounts of iron, magnesium, manganese, phosphorus, potassium, selenium, silicon, vitamin A and C, and niacin.

Ailments
Addison's Disease, Allergies, *Arthritis*, Blood Purifier, *Bursitis,* Cholesterol (reduces), Dandruff, Gallbladder, Gonorrhea, Inflammation (internal), Liver Problems, *Rheumatism*, Skin Irritations, Skin Problems, Venereal Disease.

8

HERBAL COMBINATIONS

Allergies

Function: to purify the blood, strengthen the lungs, loosen mucus and phlegm, relax the nerves and increase circulation to stimulate healing. It also provides nutrients so the body can produce natural antihistamine.

Allergies also need herbs and herbal combinations to improve *digestion*, clean and strengthen the *glands*, and nourish and fortify the *nerves*.

#1. Blessed Thistle, Yerba Santa, Scullcap and Pleurisy root.
#2. Chinese Ephedra, Senega, Golden Seal, Capsicum, Parsley, Chaparral, Althea (marshmallow) and Burdock.

Other Uses
Allergies, Asthma, Colds, Hay Fever, Mucus, Sinus, Upper Respiratory.

Anemia

Function: cleans the liver, provides rich amounts of easily assimilated iron for healthy blood, purifies the blood, tones the entire system, and eliminates uric acid from the body.

Anemia also needs herbs and herbal combinations to stimulate *circulation,* improve *digestion,* and clean and strengthen the *glands.*

#1. Red Beet, Yellow Dock, Strawberry, Chickweed, Burdock, Nettle and Mullein.

#2. Kelp, Alfalfa and Dandelion.

Other Uses
Anemia, Convulsions, Cramps, Energy, Fatigue, Kidneys, Multiple Sclerosis, Parkinson's Disease, Pituitary Gland, Senility.

Arthritis

Function: reduces inflammation and swelling, relieves tension pain, acts as a deep cleanser, neutralizes uric acid, cleans blood, stimulates circulation and heals joints.

Arthritis needs herbs and herbal combinations to improve *digestion,* clean and nourish *glands*, strengthen the *skeleton*, clean and feed the *muscles*, improve proper *circulation*, and strengthen and nourish the *nerves.*

#1. Bromelain, Yucca, Comfrey, Alfalfa, Black Cohosh, Yarrow, Capsicum, Chaparral, Devil's Claw, Burdock and Century.

Other Uses
Arthritis, Blood Cleanser, Bursitis, Calcifications, Gout, Neuritis, Rheumatism, Tennis Elbow.

Bladder and Kidneys

Function: clears mucus in bladder and kidneys, increases the flow of urine, provides antiseptic properties, strengthens and tones the urinary tract, neutralizes uric acid, soothes the nerves, cleans the blood and increases circulation.

Bladder and kidney problems need herbs and herbal combinations that will improve *digestion*, clean the *glands*, strengthen and nourish the *nerves*, and improve *circulation*.

- #1. Juniper Berries, Parsley, Uva Ursi, Dandelion and Chamomile.
- #2. Dong Quai, Golden Seal, Juniper Berries, Uva Ursi, Parsley, Ginger and Althea (Marshmallow).

Other Uses
Bed Wetting, Bladder Problems, Bloody Urine, Fevers, Diuretic, Kidney Problems, Urinary Problems.

Blood Purifier

Function: purifies the blood, detoxifies poisons, increases circulation, eliminates excess fluids, acts as a tonic, and a sedative for nervous exhaustion, glandular balance and builds the immune system.

When the blood needs cleansing, it is also vital to use herbs and herbal combinations to clean the *glands*, nourish and clean the *kidneys* and *bladder*, and make sure that the *bowels* are functioning properly.

#1. Pau D'Arco, Red Clover, Yellow Dock, Burdock, Sarsaparilla, Dandelion, Chaparral, Cascara Sagrada, Buckthorn, Peach Bark, Oregon Grape, Stillingia, Prickley Ash and Yarrow.

Other Uses

Acne, Age Spots, Arthritis, Blood Purifier, Boils, Cancer, Canker Sores, Colon, Constipation, Cysts, Eczema, Erysipelas, Eruptions, Infection, Insect Bites, Jaundice, Liver , Lymph Glands, Pancreas, Poison Ivy & Oak, Pruritus, Psoriasis, Ringworm, Rheumatism, Scurvy, Skin Problems, Spleen, Sugar Diabetes, Tetters, Tonsillitis, Tumors, Undulant Fever, Uric Acid Buildup, Venereal Disease, Worms.

Bone Combination
(Also for flesh, cartilage and connective tissues)

Function: to supply minerals (all diseases need minerals for healing), healing properties for all ailments, removes congestion, cleans blood vessels, strengthens the bones, muscles and connective tissues, strengthens the nerves and removes congestion in the blood vessels.

When any healing takes place in the body, the *glands* need to be nourished and cleansed, *circulation* and *digestion* need to be improved.

#1. Comfrey, Golden Seal, Slippery Elm and Aloe Vera. (Use internally and as poultice.)

#2. Chickweed, Alfalfa, Oatstraw, Irish Moss, Horsetail, and Valerian Root.

#3. Comfrey, Horsetail, Oatstraw and Capsicum.

#4. White Oak, Comfrey, Mullein, Black Walnut, Marshmallow, Queen of the Meadow, Chamomile, Devils' Claw, and Scullcap. (Use as poultice and tea for drinking.)

#5. An excellent combination to aid in strengthening the bones. Weakening of the bones start as early as the twenties. Calcium is necessary for bone health but other vitamins and minerals are involved in the absorption and normal bone formation:

Calcium, Magnesium, Iron, Manganese, Beta-carotene, Vitamin B6, C, Betaine HCL, Papaya Fruit, Pineapple Powder, Licorice, Root, Coix, Ma Huang, Horsetail, Valerian, Parsley, Vitamin B12 and Potassium Nitrate.

Other Uses

Aches, Allergies, Arteriosclerosis, Arthritis, Blood Clotting, Bursitis, Cartilage, "Charlie Horse", Colds, Colitis, Connective Tissues, Convulsions, Cramps, Female Problems, Flesh, Flu, Fractures, Growing Pains, Gout, Headaches, Heart Palpitations, High Blood Pressure, Hormonal Balance, Hypoglycemia, Illness, Infections, Insomnia, Joints, Lactation, Menopause, Menstrual Problems, Nerves, Osteoporosis, Pains, Pregnancy, Puberty, Rheumatism, Scoliosis, Skin Problems, Teeth, Tennis Elbows, Ulcers, Varicose Veins, Water Retention, Wounds.

Candida Combination

Function: to kill off the candida fungus and strengthen the immune system. Very useful for those on the birth control pill, on antibiotics, or other medications, allergies or a weak immune system.

#1. Acidophilus, Black Currant Oil, Vitamins A, E, C with bioflavonoids, Pantothenic Acid, Biotin, Zinc, Selenium, Caprylic Acid, Garlic, Pau D'Arco, Golden Seal, Lemon Grass, Rose Hips, Yucca.

Other Uses
Allergies, Chemical Poisoning, Frequent Illness, Infections, Immune System, Pre-Menstrual Syndrome, Weight Control.

Chelation Combination

The natural nutritional chelating elements work together in a bonding reaction by surrounding the plaque and drawing it from the veins much like a magnet attracts metal.

#1. Vitamin A, B complex, C, E, Magnesium, Manganese, Chromium, Potassium, Selenium, Choline, Methionine, Zinc, Cysteine (sulphur amino acid), Iodine, Iron, Bioflavonoids.

Other Uses
Atherosclerosis, Coronary Heart Disease, Arthritis, Heavy Metal Poisoning, Immune System, Stroke.

Cleansing Combination

A gentle cleansing combination of herbs, vitamins and minerals that works effectively and gradually to clean the body of toxins.

#1. Black Walnut, Herbal Cleansing Formula, Digestion, Combination, Psyllium, Lower Bowels Combination, Vitamins and Minerals.

Other Uses
Cell Cleanser, Constipation, Fatigue, Indigestion, Worms.

Colds and Flu

Function: to aid circulation for rapid healing, fight infection, expel mucus, purify the blood, tonic for the lungs, sooth the stomach, help to lower fevers, act as an internal antiseptic, break up congestion and strengthen the immune system..

Colds and flu also need herbs and combinations to nourish the *lungs*, feed and open the pores of the *skin*, improve *circulation*, clean and improve the *glands*, strengthen and feed the *nerves*, and make sure the *bowels* are clean.

#1. Rose Hips, Chamomile, Slippery Elm, Yarrow, Capsicum, Golden Seal, Myrrh Gum, Peppermint, Sage and Lemon Grass.
#2. Bayberry root, Ginger, White Pine Bark,Capsicum and Cloves.
#3. Garlic, Rose Hips, Rosemary, Parsley, and Watercress.

Other Uses
Asthma, Bronchitis, Childhood Disease, Circulation, Colds, Congestion, Ear Infections, Fevers, Flu, General Infections, Immune System, Mucus, Viral Infections, Tonsillitis.

Colitis

Function: helps soothe, heal and strengthen the bowels, draws out impurities, relieves gas pains, settles stomach, relaxes stomach muscles and the nerves.

Colitis and colon problems need herbs and herbal combinations to help clean and nourish the *mucous membranes, glands,* improve *digestion, circulation* and *colon* health. Also the *nerves* need to be strengthened and nourished.

> #1. Comfrey, Althea (Marshmallow), Slippery Elm, dong Quai, Ginger and Wild Yam.
> #2. Comfrey and Pepsin.

Other Uses
Bowel Problems, Colitis, Colon-irritable, Diarrhea, Indigestion, Intestinal Mucus, Mucus Cleansers, Ulcers.

Digestion

Function: to improve digestive disorders. Most ailments are improved when digestion is strengthened. These herbs help to calm a nervous stomach, aid digestion, digest proteins, prevent cancer, provide enzymes for proper digestion. They are also valuable for the digestion of proteins left in the colon.

When digestion is a problem, herbs and herbal combinations are needed to clean the *glands*, to increase *circulation*, and strengthen and nourish the *nerves*.

- #1. Papaya, Ginger, Peppermint, Wild Yam, Fennel, Dong Quai, Spearmint and Catnip.
- #2. Papaya Peppermint. (Natural acid neutralizer).
- #3. Pepsin, Pancreatic, Mycozyme, Papain, Bromelains, Bile Salts and Betaine HCI.
- #4. Hydrochloric Acid, Betaine and Pepsin. (Especially to digest protein).
- #5. Comfrey and Pepsin. (Soothes the digestive tract and dissolves mucus on the walls of the intestines.)

Other Uses
Ailments (Allergies, Bloating, Colon Cleanser, Digestive Problems, Gas (intestinal), Heartburn, Hiatal Hernia, Weight Problems).

Energy and Fitness

Function: strengthens the body, builds immunity, eliminates toxins, stimulates circulation, cleans blood, improves digestion, calms nerves, cleans glands and nourished the body.

To improve energy and fitness in the body, other herbs and herbal combinations may be beneficial in improving the *nerves*, cleaning the *colon*, and making sure there is proper *digestion*.

#1. Siberian Ginseng, Ho Shou Wu, Black Walnut, Licorice, Gentian, Comfrey, Fennel, Bee Pollen, Bayberry, Myrrh Gum, Peppermint, Safflower, Eucalyptus, Lemon Grass and Capsicum.
#2. Capsicum, Siberian Ginseng, and Gotu Kola.
#3. Mahuang, Dong Quai, Ho Shou Wu, Huang Chi, and Siberian Ginseng.

Other Uses
Diets, Drug Withdrawal, Endurance, Energy, Exhaustion, Fasting, Fatigue, Glands, Longevity, Memory, Pick-up, Senility.

Endurance

Function: strengthen mental anxiety and nerves, acts as a tonic for the endocrine glands, builds stamina and resistance to disease, burns off excess toxins and fatty material, balances sugar levels, supplies energy, strengthens the whole system, increaases circulation, and aids digestion. Rejuvenates the adrenal glands, stimulates liver and gall bladder. Contains antiseptic properties to disinfect germs. A combination to help fortify the immune system.

When the body needs to develop endurance, herbs and herbal combinations that aid other areas of the system are needed. *Digestion* needs improving, more *circulation* is needed for nutrients to assimiliate, the *glands* need to be cleaned and nourished, and the *nerves* need to be fed and strengthened.

#1. Siberian Ginseng, Ho Shou Wu, Black Walnut, Licorice, Gentian, Comfrey, Fennel, Bee Pollen,

Bayberry, Myrrh, Peppermint, Safflower, Eucalyptus, Lemon Grass and Capsicum.

Other Uses
Aging, Athletic Endurance, Diets, Endurance, Energy, Fasting, Fitness, Glands, Strength.

Eye Problems

Function: strengthens the eys, draws out toxins, kills infections, contains healing properties, and improves circulation in eye area.

Also herbs and herbal combinations are needed that aid *circulation*, improve *glands*, and strengthen *nerves*. The *mucous membranes* need to be cleaned and nourished.

#1. Golden Seal, Bayberry and Eyebright.
#2. Golden Seal, Bayberry, Eyebright, Red Raspberry and Capsicum. The tea is steeped and strained will before rinsing the eyes.

Other Uses
Air Pollution, Allergies, Cataracts, Conjunctivitis, Diabetes, Eye Inflammations, Glaucoma, Hay Fever, Itching, Styes, Vision (improves).

Fasting or Dieting

Function: to strengthen the body while fasting or dieting. Burns excess fat, nourishes glands, calms the nerves, acts as internal antiseptic, elminiates mucus, and cleans liver and veins.

When fasting and dieting, other parts of the body need to be strengthened. Herbs and herbal combinations are needed to aid better *digestion*, clean and nourish the *glands*, improve overall *circulation*, nourish and strengthen the *nerves* and make sure the *colon* is working properly.

#1.   Licorice, Hawthorn, Fennel, and Red Beet.

Other Uses
Adrenals (supports), Dieting, Fasting, Heart, Liver.

Female Problems

Function: helps balance hormones, reduces swelling, provides minerals and vitamins, acts as a nerve relaxant, neutralizes uric acid, contians diuretic properties, prevents hemorrhage, tranquilizes central nervous system, regulates menstruation, and nourishes female and adrenal glands. Helps in digestion and circulation.

It is important to make sure that *digestion* is functioning properly, that the *nerves* are strengthened and nourished with nervine herbs, and that the *glands* are cleaned and stimulated with jumping on the trampoline. *Circulation* needs to be improved.

#1.   Red Raspberry, Dong Quai, Ginger, Licorice, Black Cohosh, Queen Of the Meadow, Blessed Thistle, and Marshmallow.
#2.   Golden Seal, Red Raspberry, Black Cohosh, Queen of the Meadow, Althea (marshmallow), Blessed Thistle, Dong Quai, Capsicum and Ginger.

#3.   Golden Seal, Capsicum, False Unicorn, Ginger, Uva Ursi, Cramp Bark, Squaw Vine, Blessed Thistle, and Red Raspberry.

Other Uses
Breast Problems, Cramps, Hormone Balance, Hot Flashes, Hysterectomy, Menopause, Menstrual Prblems, Morning Sickness, Sterility, Uterine Infections, Vaginal Problems

General Cleanser

Function: to help clean the whole system. It cleans and purifies the blood, provides minerals to strengthen the body, kills toxins, nourishes pituitary gland, loosens mucus from the lungs, dissolves hardened mucus, kills infections, strengthens and adrenals, dissolves cholesterol, eliminates gastric disorders, stimulates circulation, improves liver function, cleans all glands, kills parasites and eliminates toxins.

When the whole body needs cleansing, it is essential to use herbs and herbal comnbinations to improve the *urinary tract,* the *colon*, and improve *digestion.*

#1.   Gentian, Irish Moss, Cascara Sagrada, Golden Seal, Comfrey, Fenugreek, Safflower, Myrrh, Yellow Dock, Echinacea, Black Walnut, Barberry, Dandelion, Buchu, Chickweed, Catnip and Cyani flowers.

Other Uses
Arthritis, Cancer, Colon, Constipation, Cysts, Diseases, Pain, Parasites, Skin Problems, Toxic Wastes, Tumors, Worms.

Glands

Function: provides natural iodine which strengthens and reactivates the glands, builds the nerves and cleans the blood. Increases activity of the liver, and provides essential minerals for healthy glands.

Herbs and herbal combinations are also needed to clean the *glands,* increase *circulation*, build the *nerves* and improve proper *digestion*. It is also essential to improve *colon* function for eliminating waste material.

    #1. Kelp, Dandelion and Alfalfa.

    #2. Kelp, Irish Moss, Parsley, Hops and Capsicum.

Other Uses
Asthma, Breasts, Bronchitis, Croup, Liver, Lymph Congestion, Mucus, Nerves, Pain, Pets (Vitamin and Minerals), Pituitary, Pleurisy, Pneumonia, Rheumatism, Thyroid, Tonsillitis, Tuberculosis.

Glandular Combinations
Ovaries (Female)   Prostate (Male)

Function: to give nutritional support to the body's glands and organs. They contain extracts from the pituitary, adrenal, thymus, pancreas, kidney, heart, brain and spleen. The female contains ovarian extract and the male contains prostate extract.

Other Uses
Female Problems, Hormonal Imbalance, Male Problems.

Hair, Skin and Nails

Function: to provide minerals and vitamins and necessary for healthy skin, hair and nails. Helps to prevent falling hair, stimulates hair growth, acts as an astringent to tone the scalp and stimulates the skin function.

For proper nourishment of hair, skin and nails, it is necessary to use herbs and combinations to clean and nourish the *glands*, increase *circulation*, strengthen the *nerves* and improve *digestion*.

#1. Dulse, Horsetail, Sage and Rosemary.
#2. Kelp, Dandelion and Alfalfa.

Other Uses
Anemia, Hair, Infertility, Mineral Balance, Nails, Pregnancy, Skin.

Heart and Blood Pressure

Function: feeds and strengthens the heart, helps to prevent blood clots near heart, rich in minerals for the heart and blood, improves circulation, lowers blood pressure, kills infections and cleans the blood vessels. Also equalizes blood pressure.

To improve heart and blood pressure, it will help to use herbs and herbal combinations to strengthen the *nerves*, clean and nourish the *glands,* and feed and strengthen the *bones, flesh, cartilage,* and *connective tissues*

#1. Hawthorn, Capsicum and Garlic.
#2. Capsicum, Garlic and Parsley.

Other Uses
Adrenals, Arteriosclerosis, Anxiety, Circulation, Cholesterol, Fatigue, Hardening of Arteries, Irregular Heart Beat, Liver, Pain, Shock, Varicose Veins.

Hypoglycemia

Function: supplies energy to a weakened system, helps the adrenal glands to produce more adrenalin and encourages the pancreas to manufacture natural insulin. Cleans the liver and eliminates acids in the blood, and stimulates and cleans the system

Hypoglycemia needs herbs and herbal combinations to clean and strengthen the *glands*, increase better *circulation,* improve *digestion* and strengthen and feed the nerves.

#1. Licorice, Safflower, Dandelion and Horseradish

Other Uses
Adrenal Glands, Anemia, Energy, Liver, Pancreas, Weakened System.

Immune Combination

There are certain nutrients that have been found to protect the immune system. A healthy immune system is the key to preventing illness.

#1. Vitamin A (beta carotene), C, E, Selenium, Zinc, Barley Juice Powder, Wheat Grass Juice Powder, Cabbage Powder, Broccoli Powder, and Asparagus Powder.

Infections

Function: to purify the blood and increase resistance to infections. Eliminates toxic waste, equalizes circulation, and strengthens the whole system. Acts as a natural antibiotic to kill bacteria and virus without side effects. Stimulates the body to heal itself. Number one is used for hypoglycemia because Golden Seal can lower blood sugar in some people.

Infections need herbs and herbal combinations that improve the health in the *muscles, connective tissues, bones* and *cartilage*--also *nerves* and *circulation.*

- #1. Echinacea, Yarrow, Myrrh and Capsicum.
- #2. Echinacea, Golden Seal, Yarrow, and Capsicum.
- #3. Golden Seal, Black Walnut, Althea (marshmallow), Echinacea, Plantain and Bugleweed.

Other Uses
Breast (infection), Colds, Contagious Disease, Earache, Fevers, Flu, Gangrene, Glands (Infected and Swollen), Infections, Lungs, Measles, Mononucleosis, Mumps, Rheumatism, Scarlet Fever, Sinus Infection, Throat (sore), Tonsillitis, Typhoid Fever.

Insomnia

These herbs contain natural tranquilizing properties that leave you with a refreshed feeling. Acts as a relxant, sedative and tonic. Feeds the nerves, controls nervous disorders, and relaxes the mind. Helps to produce natural sleep, helps in restlessness, and acts as a nervine for insomnia.

Herbs and herbal combinations are also needed to clean and nourish the *glands*, and to make sure there is proper *digestion* and assimilation of the nutrients.

    #1.   Valerian, Scullcap and Hops.

Other Uses
Convulsion, Headaches, Hyperactivity, Nerves, Palsy, Relaxant, Stress.

Liver and Gall Bladder

Function: helps correct liver disease, provides nutrients for healthy liver function, detoxifies poisons, clears liver obstructions, aids in circulation, natural diuretic, provides vitamins and minerals for healthy organs, heals damaged liver, stimulates liver bile, acts as a tonic for mental and physical harmony, aids digestion and strengthens the whole system.

When the liver and gall bladder are in trouble, herbs and herbal combinations should be used to nourish and clean the *glands, blood*, increase *circulation*, feed and strengthen the *muscles.*, feed the *nerves* and make sure there is proper *digestion* and assimilation.

#1. Red Beet, Dandelion, Parsley, Horsetail, Liverwort, Black Cohosh, Birch, Blessed Thistle, Angelica, Chamomile, Gentian and Golden Seal.

#2. Barberry, Ginger, Cramp Bark, Fennel Seed, Peppermint, Wild Yam and Catnip.

Other Uses
Age Spots, Cleansing, Gall Bladder, Kidneys, Panceas, Spleen.

Lower Bowels

Function: helps restore tone to a relaxed bowel, cleans and nourishes the system, stimulates bile function, helps in constipation, is calming to the gastrointestinal tract, supplies energy, is beneficial to the liver, stimulates the bowels, settles the stomach, contains antibiotic properties, cleans the urinary tract, is a natural diuretic, cleans mucus from the system, fights infections, is rich in iron and other essential minerals.

When the bowels are in trouble the *glands* also need cleansing, *circulation* needs to be improved, and the *skin* along with the mucous membranes needs to be functioning properly.

#1. Cascara Sagrada. Buckthorn, Licorice, Capsicum, Ginger, Barberry, Turkey Rhubarb, Couch Grass and Red Clover.

#2. Dong Quai, Cascara Sagrada, Turkey Rhubarb, Golden Seal, Capsicum, Ginger, Baberry, Fennel, and Red Raspberry.

Other Uses
Bad Breath, Bowel Discomforts, Cleansing, Colitis, Colon, Constipation, Croup, Diarrhea, Intestinal Mucus, Parasites.

Lungs

Function: removes mucus, helps lower fevers, heals inflammation of tissues, heals and restores new cell tissues, has antibiotic properties for upper respiratory system, coats and soothes the membranes as they heal, and calms and feeds the nerves.

More help is usually needed when there are lung problems. Special emphasis should be on strengthening and feeding the adrenals, colon, and the kidneys. When the kidneys are not doing their job of cleaning, the lungs try to do it for them. Herbs and herbal combinations to help in better *circulation*, to build the *nerves*. The *glands* usually need to be cleaned along with the *mucous membranes* and the *colon*.

#1. Comfrey and Fenugreek.
#2. Marshmallow, Chinese Ephedra, Mullein, Lady's Slipper, Catnip, Senega, and Slippery Elm.

Other Uses
Allergies, Asthma, Bronchitis, Coughs, Croup, Emphysema, Hay Fever, Lung Congestion, Mucus, Pneumonia, Sinus Problems, Upper Respiratory System.

Menopause

Function: proves nutrients so the body can produce natural estrogen, helps hot flashes, and acts as a sedative to contract the uterus. Stimulates adrenal glands, supplies energy, stimulates reproductive organs, headaches and depression. Corrects hormonal imbalances, and stimulates progesterone and cortin to achieve glandular balance.

Menopause is the time when more herbs and herbal combinations are needed to build up the *nerves*, increase *circulation* (both with exercise and internally), and the *glands* need to be fed and cleaned. *Digestion* is one of the most imporant functions that needs to be working as we age.

#1. Black Cohosh, Licorice, False Unicorn, Siberian Ginseng, Sarsaparilla, Squaw Vine and Blessed Thistle.

Other Uses
Hormone Imbalance, Hot Flashes, Gland Malfunctioning, Menstrual Problems, Morning Sickness, Sexual Impotence, Uterus Problems.

Nerve and Relaxant

The nervine herbs are useful in almost all ailments. The nervine herbs are an important part of a diet to build the immune system. The nervous system is connected to the immune system. These combinations provide properties for the nervous disorders, pain relievers, tones and feeds the nerves, natural tranquilizers, contains B vitamins for the nerves, cleans the system, has soothing effect on the nervous system, increases circulation (circulation is essential for healing) in effected area, and eliminates toxic wastes. Acts as a tonic for an exhausted nervous system and is calming to the body and mind.

The nerves also need herbs and herbal combinations to strengthen the *glands* and improve *digestion.* More *circulation* to the system increases healing.

#1. White Willow, Black Cohosh, Capsicum, Valerian, Ginger, Hops, Wood Betony and Devil's Claw.

#2. Black Cohosh, Capsicum, Valerian, Lady's Slipper, Passion Flower, Scullcap, Hops and Wood Betony.

Other Uses
Arthritis, Asthma, Convulsions, Cramps, Gargle, Headaches, Hyperactivity, Hypoglycemia, Hysteria, Insomnia, Nervous Disorders, Nightmares, Muscular Pain (external), Shock, Stress.

Pain

Function: provides natural nutrients to calm the nerves, stops pain, feeds the nervous system, cleans the body, provides circulation (circulation helps in pain), and strengthens the nervous system.

Pain in the body also needs herbs and herbal combinations to nourish the *muscles, connective tissues* (need minerals in these areas). The *glands* need to be cleansed and nourished, and also the *liver, kidneys* and *colon.*

#1. Valerian, Lettuce Leaves, Capsicum and White Willow Bark.
#2. DL-Phenylalanine and L-Tryptophan in herbal base containing Pau D'Arco, Valerian, Chinese Ephedra, Dandelion and Hops.

Other Uses
Afterpain, Arthritis, Bronchitis, Cramps, Fevers, headaches, Heartburn, Mucus, Muscular Pain, Sinus Congestion, Toothache, Worms.

Pancreas and Diabetes

Function: stimulates natural insulin in the body, regulates sugar in the blood, feeds the glands, builds resistance to disease, helps restore function of the pancreas, contains antibiotic properties, nourishes the body, calms the nerves, soothes and heals all parts of the body, and stimulates cell growth and activity.

Herbs and herbal combinations are needed to strengthen and nourish the *nerves*, clean and nourish the *urinary tract*, make sure *digestion* is functioning in the system, improve *circulation* and make sure the *glands* are in working order.

#1. Golden Seal, Juniper Berries, Uva Ursi, Huckleberry, Mullein, Comfrey, Yarrow, Garlic, Capsicum, Dandelion, Marshmallow, Buchu, Bistort and Licorice.
#2. Cedar Berries, Uva Ursi, Licorice, Capsicum, Mullein and Golden Seal.

Other Uses
Adrenal Glands, Bladder, Blood Sugar Problems, Diabetes, Gall Bladder, Fasting, Glucose Intolerance, Hyperglycemia, Glycosuria (sugar in urine), Hypoglycemia, Kidneys, Liver, Pancreas, Spleen.

Parasites and Worms

Function: expels worms and parasites, provides nutrients, tones the liver, cleans deeply into the system where only the blood and lumphatic fluids penetrate, heals and nourishes the system, stimulates natural activity of the colon, stops internal bleeding, soothes inflamed and irritated nerves, helps bleeding bowels and draws out impurities.

When parasites and worms are in the body, herbs and herbal combinations are essential to regulate *colon* health, provide proper *digestion,* improve *circulation,* clean and nourish the *glands,* feed and nourish the *kidneys* and *liver*, and strenghten and feed the *nerves.*

> #1. Pumpkin Seeds, Culver's Cascara Sagrada, Digenea Algae, Althea (Marshmallow), Witch Hazel, Mullein, Violet and Slippery Elm.

Other Uses
Bowel (cleans), Cancer, Cleansing, Colon Cleanse, Constipation, Diabetes, Parasites, Prostate, Skin Problems, Tumors, Toxins (removes), Worms,

Potassium

This combination is important for many ailments. Potassium is essential to prevent the cells from leaking. When the cells are invaded by germs or foreign materials it can cause allergies, weak heart, lung problems and ailments of all kinds.

> #1. Kelp, Dulse, Watercress, Wild Cabbage, Horseradish and Horsetail.

Other Uses
Allergies, Regulates Bowels, Congestive Heart Failure, Colds, Constipation, Colic, Diarrhea, Diets, Fevers, Flu, Fractures, Glands, Heart Problems, Hypertension, Hypoglycemia, Insomnia, Nervousness, Regulates Acid and Alkaline Balance, Severe Injuries (like burns), Water Retention, Weight Control.

Prenatal

Function: to control hemorrhaging, nervousness and help in delivery pains. It reduces high blood pressure, strengthens the veins, strengthens the uterus in childbirth, provides minerals for healthy baby and mother, and aids in easy labor while relieving pain.

During pregnancy the *glands* need to be kept clean and free from toxins, the *nerves* need strengthening because of the stress on the body, *digestion* is essential for the proper assimilation of nutrients, *circulation* and the *colon* must be in good working order.

> #1. Black Cohosh, Squaw Vine, Dong Quai, Butcher's Broom and Red Raspberry.

Other Uses
*Childbirth, Menstrual Cramps, Uterus (strengthens),
Deliver, Hormone Regulator.*

Pre-Menstrual Combination

A combination of vitamins, minerals and herbs for
women of any age to provide nutritional support for a
healthy menstrual cycle and during menopause.

#1. Contains Chinese Herbs including: Dong Quai,
     Peony, Bupleurum, Hoelen, Atrcylodes,
     Codonopsis, Alisma, Licorice, Magnolia,
     Ginger, Peppermint, Moutan, Gardenia, and
     Eyperus. Also contains Vitamin A, (beta
     carotene), D, B1, B2, B6, B12, C, Niacinamide,
     Pantothenic Acid, Folic Acid, Biotin, Choline,
     Calcium, Magnesium, Iodine, Potassium, Iron,
     Copper, Zinc, Manganese, Potassium,
     Selenium, Chromium and Vitamin E. Also
     contains Alfalfa, Bee Pollen, Golden Seal,
     Myrrh Gum, Chamomile, Psyllium, Rose Hips,
     Dandelion.

Other Uses
*Hormonal Imbalance, Menopause, Menstrual Problems,
Pre-Menstrual Syndrome.*

Prostate

Function: stimulates secretion of the liver, kidneys
andlymph glands, expels mucus, acts as a diurectic,

supplies energy, stimulates natural cortisone production, relieves inflammation and reduces pain of swollen glands, helps to balance hormones, contains antibiotic and antiseptic properties, and eliminates toxins from the bladder. Very rich in vitamins and minerals.

Prostate problems also need more help in the *muscles* and *connective tissues* of the body, also the *nerves* need to be strengthened and nourished.

#1.   Black Cohosh, Licorice, Kelp, Gotu Kola, Golden Seal, Capsicum, Ginger, and Dong Quai.

#2.   Cedar Berries, Golden Seal, Capsicum, Parsley, ginger, Siberian Ginseng, Uva Ursi, Queen Of The Meadow and Marshmallow.

Other Uses
Bladder, Hormone Regulator, Kidneys, Liver, Spleen, Urinary Tract.

Sex Rejuvenation

Function: to help correct impotence, stimulate body energy, and provide circulation for the heart and all parts of the body. It is an excellent blood purifier, and increases the body's resistance to infections. Helps to balance hormones (both male and female), increases sperm count in the male and strengthens the eggs in the female. Provides vitamins and minerals to the body.

For problems with hormone imbalance in male and female, make sure that *digestion* is functioning, that the *nerves* are fed and nourished, and that the urinary tract is kept in good working order. All the *glands* need to be fed and cleaned.

#1. Siberian Ginseng, Echinacea, Saw Palmetto, Gotu Kola, Damiana, Sarsaparilla, Zinc Gluconate, Garlic, Capsicum and Chickweed.

Other Uses
Energy, Frigidity, Hormone Balancer, Hot Flashes, Impotence, Longevity, Menopause, Senility, Sex Stimulant, Sterility.

Stress Combination

A nutritional combination to calm and nourish the nerves and feed the central nervous system. It provides the body with the nutrients necessary to meet every day stresses.

#1. Contains Schizandra, Vitamin C with Bioflavonoids, B1, B2, B6 (same amount of each), Pantothenic Acid, Folic Acid, B12, Biotin, Choline and Inositol. Contains Bee Pollen, Valerian, Scullcap, and Hops.

Other Uses
Allergies, Nervous Disorder, Nutritional Deficiencies, Exhaustion, Stress.

Thyroid

Function: purifies and strengthens the cellular structure and vital fluids of the system, promotes glandualr health, Rich in minerals, strengthens the tissues in the brain and heart, burns up excess toxins, builds resistance to infections and disease, helps to regulate metabolism, and is valuable in glandular balance.

Thyroid problems also need help in *circulation,* (physically and internally). The *nerves* also need to be properly cared for with nervine herbs to nourish and strengthen function.

   #1. Irish Moss, Kelp, Black Walnut, Parsley, Watercress, Sarsaparilla and Iceland Moss.
   #2. Kelp, Irish Moss, Parsley, and Capsicum.

Other Uses
Good for all ailments to support the body when under stress; Allergies, Digestion, Energy, Epilepsy, Fatigue, Glands, Goiter, Hormones, Lymphatic System, Water Retention, Weight Control.

Ulcers

Function: speeds the healing of ulcers, strengthens the digestive system, prevents and stops internal bleeding, eliminates toxins from the stomach and colon, and provides vitamins and minerals to strengthen the whole system.

When ulcers are present it is important to keep the *skin* brushed and cleaned so the pores can do the job of eliminating toxins. The *mucous membranes* need to be fed and nourished. All the *glands* and *nerves* need to be fed and cleansed for proper healing of ulcers.

#1.   Golden Seal, Capsicum and Myrrh.

Other Uses
Bad Breath, Canker Sores, Colitis, Colon, Diverticulosis, Dysentery, Heartburn, Hiatal Hernia, Indegstion, Mouth Sores, Stomach Ulcers.

Weight Control Aids

Function: dissolves fat in the blood vessels; purifies the liver and blood; provides potassium to eliminate food craving, gives energy boost, counteracts stress; acts as a digestive aid; helps produce more adrenalin, cleans lymphatic glands, burns excess toxins, feeds the brain to provide strength, supports the heart and circulation and helps in water retention.

To provide complete help for weight control the *nerves* need to be nourished and strengthened, the *muscles* and *connective tissues* need minerals (calcium, silicon, phosphorus and natural sodium) to prevent imbalances of toxic materials. The *glands* need to be kept cleaned and fed for the proper balance of body weight.

#1.   Chickweed, Cascara Sagrada, Licorice, Safflower, Echinacea, Black Walnut, Gotu Kola, Hawthorn, Papaya, Fennel and Dandelion.

Other Uses
Constipation, Digestion, Energy & General Cleanser, Glands, Water Retention.

Weight Control Kit

Instant Protein Drink--complete protein with all the essential amino Acids for tissue repair. Herbal combination containing Vitamin B6, Lecithin, Chickweed, Cascara Sagrada, Senna, Kelp, Cider Vinegar and Licorice Root.

Vitamin and Mineral Combination--natural combination of multi-vitamins and minerals. Also contains Linseed Oil Capsules.

9

AMINO ACIDS

Amino acids are the nucleus of every living cell. They are the basis of life itself. In nutritional research they have been very much overlooked or neglected, but today amino acids in their proper balance are being recognized as a great power in restoring and maintaining good health. A pharmacist, Robert Garrison, Jr. R. Ph. M.A. said, "As a pharmacist, let me assure you that the amino acids are far safer as therapeutic agents than most prescription drugs."

Essential and non-essential amino acids can be misleading because all are necessary. Most of the 22 identifiable amino acids can be manufactured by the body. Eight cannot and must be supplied by the diet. They are isolecine, leucine, lysine, methionine, phenylalanine, threonine, tryptopphan, and valine. The other amino acids--cysteine and tyrosine--should be classifed also as essential as they are derived from the essential methionine and phenylalanine, Also the non-essential amino acids histidine and arginine should be considered essential during the growth period as they cannot be made by the body fast enough to meet the requirements of the rapid growth of young children.

Isoleucine

Function: Essential in hemoglobin formation--lacking in the mentally and physically ill. Deficiency affects mental retardation glycine production--essential for growth and chronic disease. Used to synthesize non-essential amino acids, maintains correct nitrogen levels, regulates the function of the thymus, spleen and pituitary glands.

Sources: Beef, chicken, fish, soy protein, soybeans, eggs, liver, cottage cheese, baked beans, milk, rye, almonds, pumpkin seeds, sesame seeds, sunflower seeds, lentils, avocados, apples apricots, dates figs, bananas, papayas, peaches, pears, persimmons, strawberries. All vegetables except celery, lettuce, radishes, carrots, kale.

Leucine

Function: Necessary for growth; stimulates brain functions; compliments the function of isoleucine, essential for blood development, regulates digestion and metabolism, assists the functions of the glandular system, increases muscular energy levels.

Sources: Beef, chicken, soybeans, fish, cottage cheese, eggs, baked beans, liver, whole wheat, brown rice, almonds, brazil nuts, pumpkin seeds, lima beans, chick peas, lentils, corn, apples, apricots, dates, figs, peaches, pears, persimmons, strawberries, tomatoes, bananas, papayas.

Lysine

Function: Found to have therapeutic effects on viral related diseases, essential to adequate absorption of calcium and the formation of collagen necessary to bone, cartilage and connective tissue. Before lysine can be utilized in the formation of collagen it needs vitamin C. Without vitamin C or adequate protein to supply the amino acid lysine, wounds would not heal properly and we would be more susceptible to infection. This shows us the fascinating interrelationship of the various nutrients. Lysine strengthens the circulatory system and maintains normal growth of cells. Controls acid alkaline balance, building blocks of blood antibodies; may lessen incidence of certain kinds of cancer, regulates the pineal and mammary glands and functions of gall bladder. Necessary for all amino acid assimilation, and assists storage of fats.

Therapeutic Uses: Inhibits virus infictions when used with vitamins C, A, and zinc; controls Herpes Simplex I and II, cold sores, fever blisters, osteoprosis, rickets, dental caries, digestion.

Sources: Fish, chicken, beef, lamb, milk, cheese, beans, brewer's yeast, mung bean sprouts, cabbage, carrots, beets, cucumber, celery, kale, turnip greens, alfalfa, soybean sprouts, papayas, apples, apricots, pears, grapes, most nuts, avocados, bananas, cantaloupes, dates, figs, grapefurit, oranges, peaches, pears, persimmons, strawberries, tomatoes.

Methionine

Function: Essential to prevent excessive accumulation of fat in liver; controls fat level of blood; increases production of lecithin; helps prevent cholesterol buildup; is necessary for hemoglobin development. Contains sulphur to keep hair, skin, nails and joints healthy, selenium to protect against cancer; protects against free radicals, slows down aging process, with choline protects against tumor growth, helps kidneys stay healthy.

Therapeutic Uses: Rheumatic fever, aids toxemia in pregnancy, promotes digestion, protects against ammonia rash and blisters. Bottle fed babies have high ammonia content in urine not often found in breast fed babies, methionine is the antidote. Antifatigue agent, antistress, calcms nerves, detoxifies heavy metals, histamine, prevents atherosclerosis.

Sources: Chicken, beef, fish, ham, eggs, cottage cheese, liver, sardines and milk.

Natural Sources: Brussels sprouts, cabbage, cauliflower, kale, pineapples, apples, brazil nuts, filberts, soybeans, lima beans, seeds, nuts, beans with rice, lentils with rice, avocados, bananas, cantaloupes, dates, figs, oranges, papayas, peaches, pears, persimmons, strawberries, tomatoes.

Phenylalanine

Function: Remarkable therapeutic propeties. Essential for production of adrenalin. Enhances vitamin C absoprtion and needs vitamin C and B6 for its metabolism. Necessary for thyroid gland to secrete the iodine rich hormone thyroxine to regulate the metabolic rate--(how fast food is burned). Necessary for growth and formation of skin, hair pigment--(melanin). Aids in waste elimination of kidneys and bladder. Being investigated as a useful agent in treating mental disorders.

Therapeutic Uses: Arthritis, migraine, low back pain, whiplash, AIDS, PMS, Parkinson's disease, improves immune system, appetite suppressant, diet aid, outstanding stimulant, healthy blood vessels, eye problem protection.

Sources: Beef, poultry, fish, eggs, cottage cheese, milk, most green vegetables, carrots, beets, tomatoes, pineapples, apples, most nuts, all grains, seeds, all legumes, soybeans, persimmons, strawberries, peaches, pears, apricots.

Threonine

Function: Improves assimilation and absorption of food. Essential in mental illness prevention and treatment. Required for new cell development. Works in combination with other amino acids to improve nutrient absoprtion, prevents fat build-up in liver when choline is deficient in diet; important constituent of collagen, enamel and protein.

Therapeutic Uses: Mental illness, personality disorders.

Sources: Apples, apricots, dates, figs, peaches, pears, persimmons, strawberries, tomatoes, carrots, alfalfa, green leafy vegetables, papayas, most nuts, seeds, fish, chicken, beef, soybeans, liver, eggs, beans, milk.

Tryptophan

Function: Essential for growth of body and cell tissues. Necessary for hair and skin health. Regulates sleep and mood patterns, assists in production of gastric juices, improving digestion, blood clotting, involved in chemical messages (serotonin) from brain to the pituitary gland; enhances immune system. B6 needed to catalyze tryptophan. Niacin and vitamin E enhance and keep it in bloodstream.

Therapeutic Uses: Aids in psychiatric problems, soothes nerves, insomnia, pain reliever, antidepressant, heart attacks, migraines, tension, allergies, induces sleep, especially effective when taken with starch or carbohydrates. Used successfully as alternate to the drug amitriptyline for depression.

Sources: Turkey meat (highest), poultry, dairy products, eggs, fish, cabbage, carrot, beet, celery, kale, snapbeans, brussels sprouts, alfalfa, turnips, most nuts, soybeans.

Valine

Function: Sparks mental vigor, muscular coordination, nervous system; necessary for glandular functions, required for normal growth of cells. Deficiency could lead to nervous disorders, fingernail biting, insomnia, poor mental health.

Sources: Apples, apricots, dates, figs, peaches, pears, persimmons, strawberries, tomatoes, all grains, legumes, nuts, seeds, carrots, turnips, kale, lettuce, parsnip, squash, celery, bets, okra, tomatoes.

Alanine

Function: Main nutritional function is in the metabolism of tryptophan and pyridoxine in which it plays an essential role. Strengthens cellular walls.

Therapeutic Uses: In hypoglycemia it may be used as a source for the production of glucose. Has a cholesterol reducing effect when in combination with arginine and glycine.

Arginine

Function: Considered an essential amino acid in the growth period as cannot be made by the body fast enough to meet the requirements of the rapid growth pattern of young children. Important to male sexual health as 80% of the male seminal fluid is made up of arginine. Detoxifies poisonous waste from blood; useful in sterility cases; supports the immune system; chelating agent for manganese; with ornithine involved in weight control, works with pituitary gland, the master gland involved in burning fat and building muscle tissue. Increases the size and activity of the thymus gland in stress and injuries, reduces atherosclerosis, controls, body cell degeneration, necessary for cell reproduction and muscle contraction, assists in nitrogen elimination.

Therapeutic Uses: Sterility, wound healing, atherosclerosis, growth.

Sources: Peanuts, peanut butter, cashew nuts, pecans, almonds, chocolate and edible seeds, exists in a free state in garlic and ginseng. Alfalfa, green vegetables, carrots, beets, cucumber, celery, lettuce, potatoes, parsnips.

Cystine/Cysteine

Function: A sulfur-containing amino acid. Essential as an antioxidant and free radical deactivator; detoxifying agent; bonds to toxic metals as copper, cadmium , lead and mercury. Stimulates body's disease fighting immune system. A powerful aid to the body against radiation, pollution and extending life span. A DNA repair aid. Protects against acetaldehyde (air and cigarette smoke). Works with vitamins C, E, A, B1, B5, B6, selenium and zinc to protect against cellular damage and improves health of hair and skin. Necessary for utiliztion of B5, supplies over 10% of insulin and aids pancreatic health. Stabilizes blood sugar and carbohydrate metabolism, with pantothenic acid used in treatment of arthritis--both osteoarthritis and rheumatoid.

Therapeutic Uses: Hair and skin, aging, cancer, cardiovascular disease, wound healing, burns, surgery, chronic bronchitis, emphysema, tuberculosis, arthritis.

Sources: Eggs, milk, beef, wheat, cabbage, onions, garlic, alfalfa, carrots, beets, cauliflower, kale, brussel sprouts, apples, currants, pineapples, raspberries, Brazil nuts, filberts.

Glutamine/Glutamic Acid

Function: With glucose is one of the principal fuels for the brain cells. Stimulates mental alertness, improves intelligence, physical equilibrium, detoxifies ammonia from brain, improves and soothes erratic behavior in elderly patients, improves ability to learn, retain and recall; helps in behavioral problems and autism in children; stops sugar and alcohol craving, IQ improvement in mentally deficient children, enhances peptic ulcer healing, epiletpic children and applied in schizophrenia and senility.

Therapeutic Uses: Autism, alcoholism, ulcers, epilepsy, schizophrenia, senility, stress, arteriosclerosis, mental problems.

Sources: The most prominent amino acid in wheat protein. Snap beans, brussels sprouts, carrots, cabbage, celery, kale, lettuce, papayas.

Glycine/Serine

Function: Essential for the synthesis of non-essential amino acids. Together with Arginine heals in trauma and damaged tissues. Utilized in liver detoxification, promotes energy and oxygen use in the cells, necessary for biosynthesis of nucleic acids as well as bile acids, gastric acid secretion enhanced, readily converted into serine which protects fatty sheaths surrounding nerve fibers.

Histidine

Function: Considered an essential amino acid in the growth period of young children; essential for the maintenance of myelin sheaths, necessary for nerve cell hearing mechanisms, effects the auditory nerve, deficiency can cause deafness, hearing loss, necessary in the formation of glycogen, a vital component of blood, involved in controlling the mucus level of the digestive and respiratory system, has a vasodilating action, good chelating agent, effective against radiation, iron or heavy metals, in allergic conditions, Histamine is released during trauma and stressful conditions causing allergies, but as the level of histidine increases, concentration of histamine decreases. Sexual stimulant along with niacin, B6. Histidine has been given to cosmonauts to protect against radiation.

Therapeutic Uses: Treatment of rheumatoid arthritis, cardiocirculatory conditions, anemia, allergies, stress.

Sources: Readily available from most protein foods, carrots, beets, celery, cucumbers, kale, turnip greens, alfalfa, apples, pineapples, pomegranates, papayas, most nuts.

Asparagine/Aspartic Acid

Function: Essential in metabolism of plants. Detoxificant of ammonia; enhances function of the liver; increases stamina and endurance in athletes, believed to be the cleaning of ammonia from the system. This causes resistance to fatigue, aids in transformation of carbohydrates into cellular energy.

Sources: Carrots, celery, cucumbers, tomatoes, turnip greens, grapefruits, apples, apricots, pineapples, watermelons, almonds. Found in abundance in plant protein and sprouting seeds.

Proline/Hydroxyine

Function: Essential for collagen formation and maintenance, readily transforms into hydroxyproline, needs vitamin C to be more effective.

Therapeutic Uses: Wound healing, cosmetic improvement of aging tissue.

Tyrosine

Function: With Tryptophan may be a better sleep aid than tryptophan alone; pigment of skin, hair melanin derived from tyrosine; therapeutically alters brain function, useful agent in treating mental illness, tyrosine has been found to be most effective where there exists a deficiency state, patients who had previously rsponded to amphetamines may respond well to tyrosine therapy. Works synergistically with glutamine, tryptophan, niacin and B6 for controlling depression, anxiety, appetite with phenylalanine for weight control. Role in function of adrenal, thyroid and pituitary glands, creates positive feelings, elevates moods, alertness, and ambition. With tryptophan, niacin, vitamin B6, hops scullcap, passion flower and valerian root aids alcoholism.

Therapeutic Uses: Slows aging of cells, high blood pressure, Parkinson's disease, muscle development, allergies, cancer, irritability, alcoholism.

Sources: Aged cheese, beer, wine, yeast, ripe bananas, avocados, alfalfa, carrots, beets, cucumbers, lettuce, kale, parsnips, asparagus, sweet peppers, strawberries, apricots, cherries, apples, watermelons, figs, almonds, pickled herring, chicken livers.

Carnitine

Function: Considerd an "accessory" nutrient. Its primary purpose is to encourage fat metabolism in the muscles and carnitine necessary for heart, tissues and other organs. Synthesized in the liver by lysine and methionine together with adequate amounts of vitamin C, B6, B3 and iron. Vitamin C essential for conversion. Need for carnitine increases with strenuous exercise. Improves fat metabolism in heart and other organs, preventing high blood fat and triglycerides levels. Men have greater need than women, possible relation to infertility via inadequate sperm motility. Essential nutrient in newborn infants.

Therapeutic Uses: Strenuous exercise, injury, sunburn, liver damage, or a calorie restricted diet, myocardial infarction, high cholesterol levels, heart muscles, irregular heartbeat, angina, blood pressure, muscular dystrophy.

Sources: Dark turkey meat, red meat. Not found in vegetable forms of protein.

Glutathione

Function: Glutathione is a tripeptide comprising the three amino-acids--cysteine, glutamic acid and glycine. Removes poisons, protects cells from destruction, fat rancidity, cleans harmful bacteria in lungs, protects against dust, builds immunity, destroys free radicals, prevention and treatment of wide range of degenerative diseases. Along with vitamin C, A, E, selenium and zinc is used to treat chronic asthma, allergies, respiratory problems, may protect against pneumonia, lead, cadmium, aluminum, mercury, liver detoxification, regression of tumor develoment.

Therapeutic Uses: Cancer preventative, alcohol damage to liver, alcohol cravings, asthma, respiratory problems.

Ornithine

Function: Works with pituitary gland, secretes large amounts of growth hormones--burning fat and building muscle tissue. Involved with arginine in weight control. Two parts of arginine to one part ornithine on an empty stomach at bedtime, works during the night to release growth hormone by pituitary gland. Vital in urea cycle.

Taurine

Function: Stimulates production of growth hormone; synthesized from methionine and cystine, necessary for brain development and function, essential for infants not breast fed, high in mother's milk, associated with zinc in eye function, controls epileptic seizures, deficiency in taurine has induced epileptic seizure, concentrated in heart, skeletal muscles and central nervous system, potent and long lasting anti-convulsive effect, used with B6 for seizure problems, normalizes balance of other amino acids which in epilepsy are thoroughly disordered as it stablizes the excitability of membranes. Regulates osmotic control of calcium as well as potassium in heart muscles; influences blood sugar levels similar to insulin. With vitamin A and E thought to be of importance in muscular dystrophy, IQ levels in Down's Syndromes have improved with taurine supplement and B complex, C & E.

Therapeutic Uses: Anticonvulsive, heart muscles, muscular dystrophy, Down's Syndrome, epilepsy.

Sources: Animal protein not found in vegetable protein. Note: Research underway to determine if taurine may be a better approach to epilepsy than such drugs as dilantin and phenobarbitol.

Vitamins and Minerals

Vitamins and minerals are a necessary addition in this book due to their rich content found in herbs, in a natural form that is easily assimilated. Vitamins and minerals are listed with the amount is in each herb as far as they have been researched. There is research being done now on the constituents of the herbs. We will find in the very near future all the rich amounts of vitamins and minerals contained in all herbs.

The herbs listed in this book can therefore be utilized as a natural source of that specific vitamin or mineral. Examples are: Alfalfa is rich in chlorophyll, therefore is beneficial in building rich blood. Aloe vera is high in vitamin C and selenium and can be useful in healing burns, wounds, etc. Bilberry is rich in manganese, which is a mineral that is essential in improving eyesight. Chamomile is high calcium and magnesium which are calming to the nerves and are excellent for menstrual problems. Devil's Claw is rich in iron and magnesium and is therefore excellent as a blood purifier and for arthritis. Dong Quai is high in vitamin E and iron and is an excellent herb for all women's problems and the lymph glands. Horsetail is rich in silicon which is essential for healthy bones. Mullein is rich in iron and is beneficial for bleeding. Passion flower is high in calcium, and therefore is calming for the nerves. Red Clover is high in many nutrients that clean and nourish the blood. Safflower is high in potassium and sodium, which are essential for a healthy stomach. Slippery Elm is high in protein which is necessary for all illnesses.

10

VITAMINS

Vitamin A

Function: Infection fighter, essential for pregnancy and lactation, protects against radiation, air pollution, development of kidney stones, night blindness, toxins in the air, aids secretion of gastric juices for protein digestion, builds bones and teeth, prolongs longevity and delays senility, maintains and repairs healthy tissue.

Therapeutic Uses: Acne, alcoholism, allergies, athletes foot, arthritis, asthma, bronchitis, hay fever, colds, diabetes, eczema, heart disease, hepatitis, migraine, psoriasis, sinusitis, stress, tooth and gum diseases.
Note: Suggested for adults with acute cases of sore throat, earaches, colds, coughs; as much as 100,000 IU daily have been safely taken. Caution must be taken, as it is possible to overdose.

Principal Sources
Foods: Fish liver oil, liver, carrots, green and yellow vegetables, eggs, fuits, dried apricots, sweet potatoes, dairy products, sweet red peppers, dried peaches.
Herbs: Alfalfa, Blessed Thistle, Capsicum, Fenugreek, Passion Flower, Parsley,

Slippery Elm, Ginseng, Scullcap, Papaya, Saw Palmetto, Rose Hips, Red Raspberry, Uva Ursi, Peppermint, Eyebright, Dandelion, Damiana, Comfrey, Catnip, Chaparral.

Vitamin A Depletors: Contraceptives, cortisone, prednisone, alcohol, estrogen, mineral oil, most drugs, coffee, air pollutants, interior lighting.

Vitamin B1 (Thiamine)
Water soluble--small amounts
stored in heart, lever and brain

Function: Called "Morale" vitamin. Essential for health of entire nervous system, for proper functioning of digestive system, aids growth of young children, assists the body to utilize energy from carbohydrate foods, needed during pregnancy and lactation and strenuous exercise. Nourishes brain, eyes, ears, hair, heart, liver, kidneys. Blood builder, maintains intestines and stomach; alleviators of pain; prevents excessive fatty deposits on wall of arteries, aids treatment of herpes, repels biting insects, protects against effects of lead.

Therapeutic Uses: Alcoholism, anemia, depression, irritability, congestive heart failure, constipation, diarrhea, diabetes, nausea, indigestion, mental illness, stress, rapid heart rate, seasickness, air sickness, beriberi, shingles.

Principal Sources
Foods: Rice bran, wheat germ, sunflower seeds,

peanuts with skin, sesame seeds, pinto white beans, dried peas, millet, pork.

Herbs: Barberry, Burdock, Kelp, Dulce, Gotu Kola, Alfalfa, Ginseng, Scullcap, Papaya, Peppermint, Spirulina, Slippery Elm, Sage, Parsley, Butcher's Broom, Feverfew.

Vitamin B1 Depletors: Negative emotions, alcohol, cooking heat, caffeine, excess sugar, stress, tobacco, surgery, raw fish and shellfish, muscle relaxants and sulfa drugs.

Vitamin B2 (Riboflavin)
Water soluble--small amounts
stored in skeletal muscles

Function: Called the "youth vitamin". Essential for proper enzyme formation, normal growth, tissue formation, metabolism of fats, carbohydrates and protein. Helps maintain good vision, skin, nails, hair. Essential for antibody formation, sodium, potassium, balance, production of red blood cells and hormones, absorption of iron, provides extra stamina and essential during periods of lactation.

Therapeutic Uses: Arteriosclerosis, baldness, cystitis, hypoglycermia, mental retardation, muscular diseases, nervous disorders, nausea in pregnancy, obesity, stress, dizziness, trembling, depression and hysteria.

Principal Sources
Foods: Dry hot red peppers, almonds, wheat germ, wild rice, mushrooms, turnip greens,

safflower seeds, millet, dried peas, white beans, parsley, kale, cashews, sesame seeds.

Herbs: Alfalfa, Barberry, Gotu Kola, Spirulina, Parsley, Kelp, Hops, Ginseng, Slippery Elm, Sarsaparilla, Papaya and Peppermint.

Vitamin B2 Depletors: Alcohol, birth control pills, coffee, radiation, tobacco, ultraviolet light, drugs, estrogen and sugar.

Vitamin B3 (Niacinamide)
Water soluble--stored in liver

Function: Assists body to perform energy producing reactions in cells. Converts amino acid tryptophan into niacin. Promotes good physical and mental health, aids in healthy skin, tongue and digestive system. Regulates levels of blood, preventing high cholesterol and high blood pressure and heart attacks. Essential for production of male and female sex hormones, helps regulate blood sugar level in hypoglycemia and eases attacks of diarrhea. Used to treat schizophrenic and autistic children.

Therapeutic Uses: Acne, baldness, diarrhea, halitosis, high blood pressure, leg cramps, migraine, night blindness, hypertension, tooth decay, poor circulation, stress, backaches, poor memory, senility and schizophrenia.

Principal Sources
Foods: Rice and wheat bran, peanuts with skin, hot red peppers, dry wild rue, sesame seeds,

sunflower seeds, brown rice, wheat and
barley, green vegetables, beans, milk, fish,
poultry.

Herbs: Butcher's Broom, Kelp, Horsetail, Hops,
Gotu Kola, Feverfew, Spirulina, Slippery
Elm, Ginseng, Sarsaparilla, Red Raspberry,
Red Clover, Peppermint, Parsley, Papaya,
Eyebright, Damiana, Barberry.

Vitamin B3 Depletors: Caffeine, antibiotics,
alcohol, sleeping pills, estrogen, excessive sugar,
refined carbohydrates, sulfa drugs.

Vitamin B5 (Panthothenic Acid)
Water soluble

Function: "Panto" means everywhere--is found in
every living cell of the body. Essential for health of
adrenal glands and hormones; needed for proper
digestion, metabolization of fats, carbohydrates and
protein, antibody formation and regulation of growth
stimulation, vitamin utilization (radiation damge),
May stimulate pituitary gland to put out natural
cortisone.

Therapeutic Uses: With calcium helps stop grinding
of teeth at night, hypoglycemia, allergies, anemia,
arthritis, asthma, diarrha, eczema, muscle cramps, loss
of hair, premature aging, respiratory infections,
Addison's disease, baldness, cystitis, diabetes,
depression, alcoholism, tooth decay, wound healing.

Principal Sources
Foods: Queen bee royal jelly, brewer's yeast,
molasses, egg yolks, soybeans, peanuts,

wheat germ, dried peas and beans, whole grains, liver.

Herbs: Barberry, Parsley, Kelp, Hops, Gotu Kola, Papaya, Peppermint, Ginseng, Slippery Elm, Spirulina.

Vitamin B5 Depletors: DMethyl bromide, insecticidal fumigant, alcohol, coffee, heat in cooking (canning), sulfa drugs, estrogen and sleeping pills.

Vitamin B6
(Pyridoxine Hydrochloride)
Water soluble

Function: Called the "vitality vitamin". Essential for conversion of protein foods into amino acids, production of antibodies, hormone adrenalin to maintain a balance of minerals, potassium and sodium for entire nervous system, formation of red blood cells, protection against effects of an aesthetics and nausea in pregnancy; prevents formation of kidney stones, converts oxalic acid into a harmless form, protects harmful effects of gamma radiation and X-rays, aids in digestion and food assimilation, helps PMS, cancer immunity, essential for adequate enzyme function, without B6 the body can barley tolerate glucose and becomes sensitive to insulin.

Therapeutic Uses: Headaches, anemia, hypoglycemia, epilepsy, insomnia, arthritis, asthma, arteriosclerosis, Parkinson's disease, cataracts, weight control, high cholesterol levels, eczema, convulsions, heart attacks.

Principal Sources
Foods: Brewer's yeast, wheat germ, blackstrap

Herbs: molasses, honey, egg yolks, liver, almonds, soybeans, carrots, kale, okra, spinach.
Herbs: Alfalfa, Slippery Elm, Spirulina, Sarsaparilla, Papaya, Parsley, Kelp, Hops, Gotu Kola, Feverfew.

Vitamin B5 Depletors: Alcohol, oral contraceptives cause severe loss; canning and roasting, alcohol, estrogen, long storage, most drugs and stress.

Vitmain B9 (Folic Acid)
Water soluble--small
amounts stored in liver

Function: Essential for entire nervous system to stimulate production of hydrochloric acid, formation of genetic cells DNA and RNA, essential for the absorption of iron and calcium with vitamin B12 and C to break down protein foods, essential for the formation of new red blood cells, production of antibodies and the maintenance of sex organs.

Therapeutic Uses: Alcoholism, anemia, arteriosclerosis, baldness, intestinal parasites, diarrhea, dropsy, menstrual problems, mental illness, fatigue, stomach and leg ulcers, stress, blood disorders.

Principal Sources
Foods: Green leafy vegetables, fresh mushrooms, sprouts, liver, kidneys, brewer's yeast, wheat germ, eggs, yogurt, soybeans.
Herbs: Barberry, Ginseng, Feverfew, Kelp, Hops,

Gotu Kola, Parsley, Peppermint, Papaya, Slippery Elm, Spirulina.

Vitamin B9 Depletors: Contraceptives, high temperatures, alcohol, coffee, stress, sulfa drugs, tobacco, estrogen, food processing, barbiturates, dilantin.

Vitamin B12 (Cobalamin)
Slightly water soluble

Function: Calcium needed for assimilation. Only vitamin which contains a mineral element--cobalt. Essential in the metabolism of carbohydrate, fat and protein, blood cell formation and bone marrow, gastrointestinal tract, needed for normal growth, healthy skin, mucus membrane and nervous system, necessary for the body's use of amino acids and vitamin D and in the utiliztion of iron. Injections of B12 have been given in the treatment of pernicious anemia as in multiple sclerosis, great improvement as well in chronic alcoholism and diabetes mellitus and osteoarthritis.

Therapeutic Uses: Fatigue, nervous irritability, poor memory, allergies, alcoholism, pernicious anemia, ulcers, bronchial asthma, angina pectoris, bursitis, epilepsy, diabetes, hypoglycemia, insomnia, obesity, shingles, stress, neuritis, mental illness, osteoporosis, bursitis, hepatitis, multiple sclerosis.
Note: As much as 1000 micrograms found to be effective in treating pernicious anemia with no ill effects.

Principal Sources
Foods: Soybeans, wheat germ, liver kidneys, meat,

fertile eggs, milk cheese, fish, whey
brewer's yeast, pork, almonds, carrots.

Herbs: Alfalfa, Ginseng, Bee Pollen, Comfrey,
Dandelion, Spirulina.

Vitamin B12 Depletors: Laxatives, alcohol, antibiotics, apsirin, diuretics, antacids, tobacco, caffeine, estrogen, sleeping pills, contraceptives, intestinal parasites, cooking.

Vitamin B13 (Orotic Acid)

Function: Effective in the treatment of multiple sclerosis, and in the use of folic acid and vitamin B12. Not enough known at this time.

Therapeutic Uses: For health of nervous system, efficient brain functioning and multiple efficiency. Deficiency may lead to liver disorders, cell degeneration and premature aging.

Principal Sources: Found in root vegetables, fruits, yogurt, and whey.

Vitamin B13 Depletors: Water and sunlight.

Vitamin B15 (Pangamic Acid)
Water soluble

Function: Improves blood circulation and body's ability to use oxygen, metabolism of protein, fat, and sugar, stimulates the glandular and nervous systems, prevents premature aging and fat particles from accumulating in the blood, assists heart muscles and healing of cuts, stabilizes emotional and mental problems, detoxifying agent, protects against carbon monoxide poisoning and possible cancer causing chemicals and pollutants; shown to be a preventive substance in the treatment of cancer.

Therapeutic Uses: High blood pressure, high cholesterol levels, rheumatism, angina, asthma, hypertension, emphysema, alcoholism, cancer, hepatitis, cirrhosis of the liver, arteriosclerosis and headaches.

Principal Sources
Foods: Brewer's Yeast, sesame seeds, whole brown rice, pumpkin seeds, apricot kernels, grains.
Herbs: Black Walnut

Vitamin B15 Depletors: Alcohol, coffee, sunlight, most laxatives and water.

Vitamin B17 (Laetrile)

Function: Very controversial vitamin. Legal only in 15 states. Contains natural cyanide used to kill cancer cells. Rejected by FDA due to its cyanide content (feel it might be poisonous). On the other hand, it is believed by others to have cancer controlling and preventive properties that literally poison the malignant cell while nourishing all the other cells. Stimulates the hemoglobin or red cell count.
Note: For more detailed information see *People's Desk Reference-Traditional Herbal Formulas*, by F.

Joseph Montagna.

Therapeutic Uses: Cancer, sickle-cell anemia.
Note: Excessive amounts can be dangerous.

Principal Sources: Almonds, apricot kernels, cherries, nectarines, peahces, plums, peas, broad beans, apples, papayas, alfalfa seeds, berries, sorghum, millet, buckwheat, alfalfa leaves.

Vitamin B17 Depletors: Alcohol, coffee.

PABA
(Para-aminobenzoic Acid)
Water soluble--stored in body tissue

Function: Essential for synthesis of folic acid, blood cell formation, protein metabolism, hair color, skin health pigmentiaon, acts as a sunscreen, health of intestines; enhances intestinal flora activity, anti-aging.

Therapeutic Uses: Eczema, parasites, nervousness, baldness, constipation, overactive thyroid, rheumatide fevers, stress, infertility.
Note: Continual high doses (over 30 mg.) can be toxic and cause depression.

Principal Sources
Food: Brewer's yeast, liver, wheat germ.
Herbs: Papaya.

PABA Depletors: Coffee, sulfa drugs, alcohol, estrogen, food processing, water.

Choline
Soluble in water

Function: Essential for healthy liver, kidneys, brain and heart. Strengthens weak blood capillaries, aids cholesterol levels of blood, assists in preventing gallstones, in digestion of all types of fatty foods, needed for storage of minerals, especially calcium and vitamin A. Promotes even distribution of fats around the body, combines with other ingredients in the liver to produce lecithin.

Therapeutic Uses: High cholesterol levels, hepatitis, arteriosclerosis, baldness, constipation, hypoglycemia, dizziness, multiple sclerosis, glaucoma, asthma, eczema, alcoholism, muscular dystrophy, heart trouble, high blood pressure, hardening of the arteries.

Principal Sources
Foods: Liver, peas, peanuts, Brewer's yeast, fish, wheat germ, lecithin, sesame seeds, egg yolks, turnip greens, string beans, spinach.
Herbs: Barberry

Choline Depletors: Water, sulfa drugs, estrogen, food processing, alcohol, excessive sugar.

Inositol
Water soluble

Function: Cleanses blood of excessive fats, assisting the action of the heart, and reducing blood cholesterol levels by producing lecithin. Stimulates digestive action, promotes hair growth, stimulates normal growth and survival of cells in bone marrow and eye membranes.

Therapeutic Uses: Baldness, constipation, eczema, heart disease, hardening of the arteries, arteriosclerosis, cirrhosis of the liver, glaucoma, obesity, gall bladder trouble.

Principal Sources: Liver, soybean, lecithin, oatmeal, molasses, cantaloupes, lima beans, oranges, wheat germ, sesame seeds, whole wheat bread, brewer's yeast.

Inositol Depletors: Caffeine, insect sprays, alcohol, sulfa drugs, water.

Vitamin C (Ascorbic Acid)
Water soluble--amount stored in adrenal cortex

Function: Called the "youth" or "stress" vitamin, helps prevent infection by increasing and speeding up activity of white blood cells, destroying all viruses and bacteria. Primary role in formation of collagen, essential for good teeth, bones, growth of children, glandular activity-especially adrenal glands, helps detoxify harmful cancer-causing substances by reinforcing the defense system; cleans blood; converts cholesterol into bile salts for prevention of gallstones, and kidney stones-absorption of iron, enables storage of folic acid. In nature Vitamin C is always in combination with bioflavonoids. Better taken in frequent small doses. Efficacy of ascorbic acid is enhanced taken with natural vitamin C. Iodine conservation, antioxidant, detoxifies drugs, protects against nitrates and nitrites.

Therapeutic Uses: Arthritis, colds, alcoholism, allergies, tonsillitis, ear infections, atherosclerosis, baldness, carbon monoxide, heavy metal poisoning,cystitis, drug addiction, hypoglycemia, heart disease, hepatitis, obesity, prickly heat, sinusitis, tooth decay, stress, asthma, radiation.

Principal Sources

Foods: Acerola cherry juice, raw hot red peppers as well as sweet red and green peppers.

Herbs: Catnip, Ginseng, Hops, Hawthorn Berries, Eyegbright, Rosehips, Parsley, Passion Flower, Juniper Berries, Lobelia, Aloe Vera, Burdock, Dandelion, Horsetail, Bayberry.

Vitamin C Depletors: Alcohol, air pollution, cigarette smoking, birth control pills, antibiotics, stress, aspirin, pain killers, diuretics, cortisone.

Vitamin D (Calciferol)
Fat soluble-stored in
skin, brain, liver, bones

Function: Essential for health of glandular and nervous system. Main function to regulate all mineral and vitamin metabolism, especially calcium, phosphorus, vitamin A, heart action, blood clotting. Produced naturally by the action of sunlight with oily substance ergosterol. In polluted areas more vitamin D is needed. Prevents colds with vitamins A and C.

Therapeutic Uses: Acne, alcoholism, rickets, colds, eye infections, tooth decay, myopia, conjunctivitis, rheumatoid arthritis, allergies, cystitis, psoriasis, stress, cramps, constipation.

Note: Toxicity--25,000 IU over an extended period of time. Synthetic vitamin D more toxic than natural.

Principal Sources:
Foods: Eggs yolks, butter, whole dried milk, fish liver, tuna, sardines, irradiated milk, spinach.
Herbs: Fenugreek, Eyebright, Alfalfa.

Vitamin D Depletors: Mineral oil, smog, barbiturates, prednisone, dilantin, sleeping pills, cortisone, anticonvulsants.

Vitamin E (Tocopherol)
Fat soluble--small amounts
stored in liver and fatty acids

Function: Vitamin A and vitamin E activate each other. Alpha Tocopherol is the most potent form of Vitamin E. Antioxidant. Essential for effective use of linoleic acid and for health of adrenal and pituitary glands. Enhances oxygenation of blood, reduces cholesterol, increases fertility and male potency, revitalizes, strengthens heart muscles. Selenium increases power of vitamin E as well as manganese necessary for vitamin E to be more effective. Helps strengthen and tone up muscles, protects lungs, may retard cancer, prevents sterility, porotects against radiation and B group vitamins from rapid oxication.

Therapeutic Uses: Healing scar tissue, burns, aging,

blood clots, heart failure repair, diurectic-blood pressure, migraine, headaches, muscular dystrophy, cold sores, coronary thrombosis, nephritis, miscarriage.

Principal Sources

Foods: Wheat germ, lettuce, watercress, spinach, oats, corn, green peas, most green leafy vegetables, vegetable oils (found in unsaturated oils from plant foods), egg yolks, peanut oil.

Herbs: Alfalfa, Blue Cohosh, Dulse, Kelp, Dong Quai, Eyebright, Spirulina, Ginseng, Scullcap.

Vitamin E Depletors: Estrogen, birth control pills, chlorine, mineral oil, heat, food processing, inorganic iron, rancid fat.

Vitamin F (Unsaturated fatty acids)
Fat soluble, small amount stored in liver

Function: Essential for healthy function of the adrenal and thyroid glands, blood coagulation, growth and respiration of organs, healthy hair and skin, and maintaining reliance and lubrication of all cells. Stimulates conversions of cartoene into the form of Vitamin A. Some protection against effects of X-rays. Best absorbed with Vitamin E.

Therapeutic Uses: Cholesterol, hardening of the arteries, blood pressure, colitis, diabetes, allergies, diarrhea, eczema, gall stones, varicose veins, nail problems, asthma, multiple sclerosis, arthritis, acne, constipation, dermatitis, common cold and obesity.

Principal Sources:

Foods: Oats, rye, nuts, avocado, fertile eggs, whole raw milk, cod liver oil, all unsaturated vegetable oils. Besides these, many known sources found especially high: Black Currant Oil, Evening Prirmose Oil, Fish Oil Lipids.

Herbs: Alfalfa, Irish Moss.

Vitamin F Depletors: Radiation, x-rays, heat, oxygen, rancid oils, unsaturated fats.

Vitamin H (Biotin)
Water soluble--stored in liver

Function: Essential for normal growth of all body tissues and cells. for mothers during pregnancy asnd time of lactation, metabolism of carbohydrates, fat, protein and utilization of B complex vitamins, maintenance of skin, hair, all secreting glands, nerves, bone marrow, male sex hormones, fatty acid production.

Therapeutic Uses: Baldness, mental depression, dermatitis, eczema, leg cramps, digestion.

Principal Sources

Foods: Brewer's yeast, egg yolks, liver, milk, wheat germ, sprouts, molasses, yogurt.

Herbs: Alfalfa, Barberry.

Vitamin H Depletors: Process of refinement as in modern cereals, antibiotics, mineral oil, raw egg whites, sulfa drugs, alcohol, estrogen, sugar.

Vitamin K
*Fat soluble small
amount stored in liver*

Function: Essential in formation of prothrombin (a blood clotting chemical), produced in the intestines of normal healthy people. Important for normal function of the heart and liver, needs bile to be utilized, protects liver against lead pollution, required for conversion of carbohydrates into glucose. With vitamin C effective in preventing hemorrhage after sugrical operations.

Therapeutic Uses: Antihemorrhagic, excessive menstrual flow, colitis, bruises, preparation for childbirth, gall stones, coronary thrombosis.
Note: Natural vitamin K is non-toxic. Synthetic can be toxic, not more than 300-500 mcg. recommended.

Principal Sources
Foods: Egg yolks, soybeans, green leafy vegetables, liver, yogurt, whole grains, legumes.
Herbs: Alfalfa, Cornsilk, Irish Moss, Kelp, Shepherd's Purse.

Vitamin P (Bioflavonids)

Function: Increases effectiveness of vitamin C, prevents and heals bleeding gums, builds immune system, stops capillary bleeding, at least 61 flavonoids in various kinds of citrus fruits, used to preserve foods especially fruits and vegetables, prevents red blood cells, and blood platelets from clumping together, anti-inflammatory activity, natural diuretic, strengthens body's defenses, helps in maintaining healthy capillaries.

Therapeutic Uses: Colds, scurvy, rheumatism, varicose veins, pneumonia, asthma, ulcers, hemorrhoids, edema, post partum bleeding, cataracts, hypertension, respiratory infection, allergies, wound healing, viral infectins, duodenal ulcers, spontaneous aborption, hemophilia, leukemia.

Principal Sources
Foods: Citus fruit pulp, grapes, rosehips, black currants, prunes, spinach, buckwheat.
Herbs: Paprika, Black Currants, Rose Hips.

Vitamin P Depletors: Smoking, apsirin, alcohol, antibiotics, cortisone, pain killers.

Vitamin T

Function: Very little know as yet on this new vitamin. Assists in normalizing blood coagulation and forming of platelets. May improve failing memory and poor concentration:

Therapeutic Uses: Anemia, hemophilia.

Principal Sources: Found in sesame seeds, tahini and egg yolks.

Vitamin U

Function: Recently discovered. High in Chlorophyll, one of the best natural medicines available.

Therapuetic Uses: Duodenal and peptic ulcers.

Principal Sources: Found in cabbage juice, sauerkraut and raw celery juice.

Vitamin U Depletors: Heat.

11

MINERALS

Calcium

Function: Essential for smooth functioning of heart muscles and muscular movements of intestines (peristaltic action) aiding digestion. To function efficiently calcium must be in combination with magnesium, phosphorus, vitamin A, C, and D as well as zinc and inositol for proper absorption, also must have acid, otherwise will collect in joints and tissues. Necessary for the formation of bones and teeth and to maintain healthy glands. Only when calcium levels are low can a virus infection occur, improves acid-alkaline balance, metabolizes iron, helps vitamin C function, protects against heavy metals and radiative material.

Therapeutic Uses: Anemia, hemophilia, healing of bones, wounds, acne, scrofula, stress, hypoglycemia, charlie horses, leg cramps, rickets, cardiovascular health, lowers cholesterol and triglycerides, aging, arthritis, asthma, hayfever, rheumatism, menstrual cramps, backache, sleeplessness, infections.

Principal Sources

Foods: Barley, kale, cereals, sesame seeds, unrefined grains, raw cheese, goat's milk, raw cow's milk.

Herbs: Alfalfa, Barberry, Bayberry, Black Cohosh, Buchu, Fennel, Eyebright, Dandelion, Damiana, Chamomile, Chickweed, Cascara Sagrada, Parsley, Horsetail, Oatstraw.

Calcium Depletors: Aspirin, chocolate, stress, lack of exercise, lack of magnesium, lack of hydrochloric acid, mineral oil, oxalic acid, phytic acid, high animal protein diet, tetracycline, table salt, excessive phosphorus.

Chlorine
(organic)

Function: Essential for the production of vital gastric juices aiding digestion, regulates heart action and normalizes blood pressure, expels waste, purifies and disinfects, fights germs and bacteria, assists liver, rejuvenates all body's skin tissue, helps regulate acid and alkalinebalance of blood and hormone distribution.

Therapeutic Uses: Tetanus, intestinal colic, injuries, burns, restlessness, sluggish liver, breast lumps, swollen glands, skin itch and rashes, pyorrhea, catarrh.

Principal Sources

Foods: Fish, raw goat's milk, raw cheeses, sardines, rye flour.

Herbs: Alfalfa, barberry, kelp.

Note: High table salt level can give excess inorganic chlorine. Inorganic destroys vitamin E and intestinal flora.

Chromium

Function: Essential for metabolism of glucose for energy and synthesis of fatty acids and cholesterol and protein, helps in blood sugar regulation, believed to help in the prevention of heart attackes.

Therapeutic Uses: Arteriosclerosis, diabetes, growth aid, hypoglycemia, pregnant women, elderly, high blood pressure, cholesterol level.

Principal Sources
Foods: Corn oil, sugar beets, molasses, spices, whole grain cereals, clams, meat, Brewer's yeast liver.
Herbs: Kelp, Licorice, Spirulina.

Chromium Depletors: Refined starches and carbohydrates, sugar.

Cobalt

Function: Essential for human nutrition; aids in the asimilation and synthesis of vitamin B12, stimulates many enzymes for the body. Essential in the building of red blood cells and other cells in the miantenance and function, cobalt must be supplied by the diet, increases assimilation of iron.

Therapeutic Uses: Pernicious anemia, nervous disorder, growth aid, heart palpitations.

Principal Sources: Raw milk, goat's milk, all sea foods, apricots, meats, liver and kidneys, oysters, clams, sea vegetation.

Herbs: Dandelion, Horsetail, Kelp, Red Clover, Spirulina.

Cobalt Depletors: Alcohol, sunlight, sleeping pills, estrogen.

Copper
(trace mineral)

Function: Copper is part of every body tissue, with manganese improves proper assimilatation of iron and formation of red blood cells, RNA production, improves digestive system, involved in formation of myelin, the protective sheath of nerve fiber, maintains muscle tone, converts amino acid tyrosine that gives color to skin and hair, sunthesizes phsopho lipids, functions with vitamin C.

Therapeutic Uses: Anemia, osteoporosis, baldness, bedsores, edema, leukemia.
Note: An excess may cause arthritis.

Principal Sources
Foods: Liver, whole grain cereals, almonds, green leafy vegetables, dried legumes, beans, seafood, blackstap molasses, organ meats, bonemeal.

Herbs: Burdock, Chickweed, Comfrey, Garlic, Eyebright, Juniper, Kelp, Spirulina.

Copper Depletors: Excessive zinc and molybdenum.

Fluorine
(Organic)

Function: Called the decay resistant element. Fluorine is essential for blood, spleen, tooth enamel, bones, skin, hair, naiels, iris. Helps prevent curvature of the spine, diseases, reduces acidity of mouth which causes tooth decay. Fluorine and sodium are two elements to enable us to utilize calcium.

Therapeutic Uses: Flu, colds, eye problems, ulcers, nervousness, stress, falling hair, helps expectant mothers, parasites, varicose veins.

Principal Sources
Foods: Raw goat's milk, avocado, cheese, cabbage, garlic, oats, brown rice, seafood.
Herbs: Alfalfa, Black Walnut, Hops, Kelp, Spirulina.
Note: Inorganic fluorine considered highly toxic.

Fluorine Depletors: Cooking Heat, refined cereals impair absorption of fluorine, sugar, aluminum, salts, fluoride.

Iron
(Organic)

Function: Called the anti-anemia mineral. Calcium and copper needed for effective iron absorption, and combines with protein forms hemoglobin, improves, protein metabolism, needed to bring oxygen to the lungs and to all the body's muscular cells, improves circulation, intensofies mental vitality, liver, kidney and heart function, digestion and elimination. Iron and oxygen promote youthfulness.

Therapeutic Uses: Dizziness, depression, headaches, anemia, heartburn, breathing difficulty, heart palpitations, alcoholism, constipation, colitis, menstruation, colds, sore throat, wound healing, diabetes, peptic ulcer, nephritis.

Principal Sources

Foods: Blackberries, cherries, dried fruits, strawberry juice, greens spinach, raw egg yolks.

Herbs: Capsicum, Butcher's Broom, Horsetail, Marshmallow, Dulse, Kelp, Uva Ursi, Sarsaparilla, Golden Seal, Fenugreek, Echinacea, Dong Quai, Dandelion.

Note: Overdose agitates body functions.
    An inorganic iron test on mice proved fatal.

Iron Depletors: Phophates, food additives, food preservatives, EDTA, tea, and coffee, excessive phosphorous, manganese.

Iodine

Function: Essential for regulating the thyroid gland, manufacturing the hormone thyroxin to control the metabolism of the body, affecting growth rate, digestion, and burning up of excess fat. Regulates cholesterol levels, prevents cretinism in newborn when taken by pregnant women, essential for energy production, prevention of anemia, necessary for lymphatic system, protects against toxins in the brain.

Therapeutic Uses: Goiter, irregular heart beat, hardening of the arteris, nervousness, irritability, obesity, low blood pressure, cretinism, angina pectoris, arterio and atherosclerosis, hyper and hypothyroidism, arthritis, hair and skin problems, catarrah, breast cancer.

Principal Sources
Foods: Seafood, garlic, onions, eggplant, mushrooms, potatoes, fish roe.
Herbs: Kelp, Dulse, Black Walnut, Spirulina.

Iodine Depletors: Heat, food processing.

Magnesium

Function: Called the anti-stress mineral. Assists in the absorption of calcium, phosphorus, sodium, potassium, B complex, C and E. Essential for formation of strong bones, teeth, lungs and all body tissues; calms nerves, promotes sleep, proper digestion, nourishes the white nerve fiber of the brain and spinal cord, protects against heart attacks, activator of enzymes, in the use of protein and vitamins.

Therapeutic Uses: Alcoholism, kidney stones, arthritis, hardening of the arteries, high blood pressure, osteoporosis, leukemia, neuritis, pain preventiona, memory, senility, irritability, acidity, sinusitis, stiff muscles, neuralgia, convuslions.

Note: 30,000 mg. may be toxic.

Principal Sources

Foods: Unpolished rice, wheat germ yellow corn meal, almonds, avocados, whole grains, greens, berries, grapefruits, barley.

Herbs: Kelp, Valerian, Stevia, Scullcap, Red Raspberry, Gotu Kola, Red Clover, Papaya, Oatstraw, Mullein, Marshmallow, Licorice, Horsetail, Fennel, Eyebright, Spirulina, Peach Bark, Chickweed.

Magnesium Depletors: Alcohol, synthetic vitamin D in excess, diuretics, coffee, tobacco, refined sugar, digitalis.

Manganese
(trace mineral)

Function: Essential for the proper function of the pituitary gland as well as the healthy function of all the body's glands, manganese is a brain and nerve food element stored in combination with lecithin, required for formation of red blood cells, regulates menstrual period, essential for expectant mothers and during lactation, good memory builder, essential for protein and carbohydrate metabolism, especially for sex hormones and improves eyesight.

Therapeutic Uses: Diabetes, asthma, muscular and mental fatigue, epilepsy, and digestion.

Principal Sources
Food: Nuts, seeds, avocados, barley, kidney beans, raw egg yolks, leaf lettuce, grapefruit, apricots.

Herbs: Eyebright, Spirulina, Sarsaparilla, Red Raspberry, Ginger, Gotu Kola, Catnip, Chickweed, Bilberry, Black Walnut, Blue Cohosh, Buchu, Uva Ursi.

Manganese Depletors: Large phosphorus and calcium intake, also high iron intake.

Molybdenum

Function: Essential for enzyme actions, believed to help prevent esophageal cancer and dental caries. Frees iron stored in liver, carrying oxygen to body cells and tissues, helps eliminate toxic nitrogen waste.

Therapeutic Uses: Anemia

Principal Sources: Buckwheat, leafy dark green vegetables, lima beans, barley, wheat, germ, meat.

Molybdenum Depletors: Copper and refined foods.

Phosphorus

Function: Vitamin D and calcium essential for proper phosphorus function. Essential for cell division and reproduction, promotes secretion of hormones and maintenance and repair of entire system, stimulates blood circulation, keeps acid out of bloodstream, provides quick release of energy, utilization of fats, proteins, carbohydrates, reduces possibility of cancerous tissue formation assists transfer of fatty acids through the body, normalizes blood pressure.

Therapeutic Uses: Blood, brain, tooth and gum disorders, backache, feebleminded, sterility, impotence, anti-aging, equilibrium and coordination of muscles.

Principal Sources

Foods: Barley, beans, fish, lentils, milk, goat's milk, rice bran, dark green leafy vegetables, cheese, pumpkin seeds, nuts egg yolks, poultry.

Herbs: Alfalfa, Bilberry, Comfrey, Garlic, Oatstraw, Peach Bark, Chickweed, Burdock, Horsetail, Fennel.

Phosphorus Depletors: Sugar, excess intake of aluminum, magnesium and iron, salts from cookware, mineral oil, tobacco.

Potassium

Function: Main healing mineral. Works together with sodium to keep acid-alkaline balance. Assists recuperative powers, strengthens heart muscles, keeps body in healthy condition, improves anti-cancer cells, repairs liver, changes glycogen to glucose, aids in waste elimination, prevents ailments.

Therapeutic Uses: Physical and mental stress, calms nerves, hardening of arteries, aging, diabetes, arthritis, rheumatism, wound healer, lymph gland congestion, heart problems, allergies, liver disease, hypoglycemia, high blood pressure, diabetes.

Principal Sources
Foods:　Potato peeling broth, bitter greens, bananas, beans, almonds, whole grains.
Herbs:　Dulse, Kelp, Irish Moss, Valerian, Stevia, Scullcap, Sage, Sarsaparilla, Safflower, Red Clover, Ginger, Peach Bark, Peppermint, Parsley, Licorice, Horsetail, Hops, Garlic.

Potassium Depletors: Cooking and Processing, alcohol, coffee, diuretics, laxatives, cortisone, excess salt, sugar heat.

Selenium

Function: Selenium works with vitamin E as an antioxidant of toxic materials and helps the body utilize oxygen, assists normal body growth, helps to prevent chromosome breakage causing birth defects.

Believed to prevent many kinds of cancer, especially breast cancer, delays the oxidation of poly-unsaturated fatty acids for elasticity of all skin tissues.

Therapeutic Uses: Premature aging, skin problems, protein deficiency diseases, birth defects, scalp problems, emphysema, high blood pressure, infertility, heart function, sexual function, menopause.

Principal Sources
Foods: Bran, whole grains, tuna fish, broccoli, onions, tomatoes, asparagus, mushrooms.

Herbs: Black Walnut, Horsetail, Hawthorn Berries, Aloe Vera, Spirulina, Slippery Elm, Ginseng, Red Raspberry, Pau D'Arco, Marshmallow, Chaparral, Catnip, Black Cohosh, Blessed Thistle, Blue Cohosh, Buchu.

Selenium Depletors: High fat intake, stress.

Silicon

Function: Silicon is dependent on fluorine. Essential for healthy hair, skin, teeth. Increases alkalinity of the body, cleansing mineral, essential for healthy blood cells and proper blood circulation, protects body against the development of cancer tissue, reinforces membrane walls, lungs, ligaments, helps retain body heat and increases vigor, energy, strength and resistance.

Therapeutic Uses: Mental fatigue, baldness, nervousness, exhaustion, poor vision, infection, depression, heart, arthritis, sexual weakness, indigestion, insomnia, schizophrenic behavior, hair loss, enlargement of liver.

Principal Sources
Foods: Oats, barley, nuts seeds, cereals, grains, rice polishings, concentrated in outer skin layer of fresh fruits and vegetables.
Herbs: Oatstraw, Eyebright, Echinacea, Cornsilk, Chickweed, Licorice, Scullcap, Horsetail, Gotu Kola, Golden Seal, Alfalfa, Burdock.

Silicon Depletors: Fats, starches and sugar.

Sodium

Function: Sodium is only valuable when it is organic and balanced. Essential for production of saliva for proper digestion of all carbohydrate food, keeps calcium in body, prevents arthritis, thickening of blood, hardening of the arteries and excess mucus. Main constituent of lymphatic system, assists in elimination of carbon dioxide waste from lungs, promotes pliable joints, essential to liver, pancreas and spleen, with potassium works to control substances in and out of each cell.
Note: When sodium is inorganic (table salt) it is harmful to kidneys, causes high blood pressure.

Therapeutic Uses: Digestion, vomiting, intestinal gas, neuralgia, rheumatism, gout, gallstones, bladder ailments, diabetes, blood clotting.

Principal Sources
Foods: Whey, black mission figs, okra and celery, watercress, goat's milk.

Herb's Alfalfa, Chickweed, Buchu, Burdock, Gotu Kola, Safflower, Sarsaparilla, Rosehips, Peppermint, Papaya, Parsley, Licorice, Dandelion.

Sodium Depletors: Diarrhea, exercise, hot climate, excess sweating and vomiting.

Sulphur

Function: Known as the beauty mnineral, growth promoter, keeps hair glossy and complexion clear, works with B complex vitamins, acts as an oxidizing agent, essential for protein absorption, counteracts acidosis, assists growth in children, normal function of heart muscles. Must be balanced with phosphorus, required for proper digestion, metabolism of carbohydrates, influences liver, promotes bile secretion, regulates nerve impulses, cell formation, essential in the stimulation of egg and sperm production, without sulphur babies could not be born or chickens hatched.

Therapeutic Uses: Degestion, blood purifier, hepatitis, dandruff, acne, depression, counteracts acidosis, maintains healthy hair, skin and nails, balances menstrual cycle.

Prinicipal Sources
Foods: Dale, cabbage, cauliflower, horse radish, brussel sprouts, watercress, chervil, parsley, celery, fish, eggs, dried beans, nuts.
Herbs: Alfalfa, Kelp, Mullein, Barberry.

Suphur Depletors: Cooking.

Vanadium

Function: Essential for proper circulation, prevents excessive cholesterol deposits in blood vessels and central nervous system. Essential in iron metabolism and helps in bone, cartilage and teeth.

Therapeutic Uses: Goiter, tooth decay, high cholesterol levels, heart attacks.

Principal Sources
Foods: Fish, seafood, soybeans, liver, meat, possible to inhale from air.
Herbs: Kelp.

Vanaduim Depletors: Food processing.

Zinc

Function: Essential for growth of children's bones and teeth. One of the main healing minerals for healthy hair and proper digestion of proteins, carbohydrates, essential for proper action of insulin, sugar conversion. Is essential for health of prostate gland, maufacturer of various male hormones and development of genital organs. Needed for action of B complex vitamins. Silicon and zinc are a valuable beauty aid promoting growth of hair.

Therapeutic Uses: Atherosclerosis, sterility, heart attacks, ulcers, diabetes, acne, dermatitis, retarded growth and fatigue, infection resistance, wound healing, inflammation, schizophrenia, DNA Synthesos, digestion, acid alkaline balance.

Principal Sources

Food: Whole grain cereals, wheat germ, wheat bran, pumpkin seeds, avocado, asparagus.

Herbs: Capsicum, spirulina, psyllium, garlic, sage, butcher's broom, lady's slipper, spirulina, eyebright, echinacea, bilberry, buchu, gotukola.

Zinc Depletors: Excessive calcium, antacids, alcohol, oral contraceptives.

12

NUTRITIONAL SUPPLEMENTS

Algin

Algin is a natural extract from kelp. It is a concentrated form of nutrient that is found very effective in eliminating the body of radioactive strontium 90. It is also beneficial to help eliminate the chemical additives that we ingest daily.

Algin grabs hold of the toxic material and excretes it out of the body. It acts like a magnet, drawing the radioactive material and other unwanted toxic waste that is harmful to the system.

This is another preventive herb that can be used daily for protection.

B-Complex with Vitamin C & Riboflavonoids

These nutrients need to be supplied each day in the diet. These are lacking in most diets. They are essential to protect the immune system and the nervous system. These are very beneficial for teenagers, especially those who are depressed, and lacking in nutrients.

Bentonite

Hydrated bentonite is a volcanic ash (clay). It has the ability to purify the blood by cleansing and enriching the system. It helps in diarrhea and constipation and acts on all organs of the body. All toxins and negative radiations are attracted to clay (a positive pole) and are eliminated out of the body. Parasitic organisms cannot proliferate in the presence of clay.

It has been used successfully in a colon cleanse program. See *Colon Cleanse The Easy Way*, by Vena Burnett and Jennifer Weiss. It has helped to eliminate viral infections, food allergies, spastic colitis, mucous colitis and food poisoning. It is an easy way to eliminate toxins from the system. Enemas are recommended when using hydrated bentonite internally.

Black Currant Oil

Black currant oil contains from sixteen to eighteen percent gammalinolenic acid. It is richer in essential fatty acids than evening primrose oil. These fatty acids need to be suppled in the diet. Researchers have discovered that those deficient in GLA are susceptible to every communicable disease that comes along. With our modern day plague (AIDS, candida, and etc.) the GLA will help protect the immune system.

It can benefit in alcoholism, allergies, arthritis, bowel problems, breast pain, brittle nails, candida, cancer, capillary fragility, cholesterol (lowers), coughs (nervous), cramps, female disorders, eczema, glaucoma, hair loss, headaches, heart ailments, high blood pressure, hyperactivity, immune system, mental disorders, multiple sclerosis, nerves, neuralgia, obesity, PMS, skin diseases, ulcers, and whooping cough.

Black Ointment

A salve for external use only. It has a strong drawing power to promote healing. It contains chaparral, lobelia, golden seal, comfrey, plantain, red clover, mullein, marshmallow, chickweed, poke root, wheat germ, olive oil, glycerine, pine gum, lanolin and beeswax.

It is used on boils, abscesses, splinters, carbuncles, felons, skin infections, skin cancer, cysts and tumors.

Chelated Cell Salts

These are easily assimilated trace minerals that have been broken down for the body to assimilate and utilize. Without minerals the body has a difficult time overcoming illness. Mineral balance in the body will balance body chemistry so it can heal itself.

They are derived from alfalfa, licorice and rose hips as well as from an ancient salt dome deposit. Chelated processed minerals absorb eighty percent better than unchelated and inorganic minerals.

These cell salts can be used for all illnesses. It will help balance body chemistry. One small mineral lacking in the body can cause an imbalance and illness.

Chinese Essential Oils

This is a formula based on an ancient combination of essential oils dating back one thousand years. It contains safflower oil, wintergreen oil, menthol, camphor and other essential oils.

It is like a first aid kit to keep with you at all times. It can be used for allergies, arthritis, burns, colds, coughs, cuts, headaches, insect bites and stings, itching, swelling, poison oak and ivy, muscle pain, sprains, stiff neck, sinus, stuffy nose, vomiting, motion sickness and can even be used to keep you awake on long distance driving.

Chlorophyll

Liquid chlorophyll is an all around food beneficial for tissue repair. It is easy to absorb and assimilate. It goes directly to the bloodstream without having to be digested and it saves energy. It contains the greatest amount of minerals of any land plant.

Chlorophyll is the green pigment that plants use to carry out the process of photosynthesis. This process absorbs the light energy for the reduction of carbon dioxide to sugars and other plant material. The liquid chlorophyll helps to neutralize some of the pollution that we eat and breathe. It strengthens the body so that it can fight pollution. Chlorophyll helps to keep calcium and other minerals in the body.

Chlorophyll is also a natural deodorizer. Use 1 teaspoon in a glass of water in the morning. Gargle with one part chlorophyll to nine parts water for sore throat, laryngitis and tonsillitis every few hours. Rinse mouth after teeth extraction. It helps purify the liver, soothes ulcer, helps catarrhal problems, helps build high blood count and feeds the organs iron and essential nutrients. It clears bowel toxins and helps in lung conditions. Increases milk production in nursing mothers, heals sores quickly, purifies body odors, helps nasal drip, soothing to hemorrhoids and many other conditions of the body.

Evening Primrose Oil

Contains essential fatty acids, which are compounds similar to essential amino acids that cannot be manufactured by the body and need to be provided in the diet. They are essential for many health functions. They are hormone-like substances that help in many functions of the body and in a variety of diseases.

It is used for alcoholism, allergies, asthma, arthritis, glaucoma, headaches, heart disease, menstruation, PMS, lowers cholesterol, multiple sclerosis, obesity, reduces blood pressure, skin and hair health, eczema and decreases hyperactivity in children. It helps in inflammatory diseases and disorders of the immune system

Fish Oil Lipids

Fish lipids are called "omega-3" fatty acids, which are unique in structure because they have large quantities of long chain polyunsaturates. They have the ability to help balance body chemistry and prevent diseases. Fish oil lipids improve the blood, heart disease and the immune system.

It will help in allergies, arthritis, asthma, glaucoma, high blood pressure, infertility, lupus, menstrual cramps, migraine headaches and possible cancer. It is felt that these unique fish lipids will help in many diseases.

Garlic Oil

Garlic is a natural antibiotic. It has the ability to destroy germs. It is beneficial for digestion, lung problems and cardiovascular diseases. It is beneficial for contagious diseases. It can be used in the ears along with lobelia extract for infections.

It can be used for cancer prevention, cramps, earaches, fungus, heart problems, indigestion, infections, mouth sores, parasites, sinus congestion, ulcers, viruses and worms--to name a few.

Glucomannan

Glucomannan can be a beneficial supplement in reducing cholesterol levels significantly by absorbing excess cholesterol and eliminating it. It works well with lecithin in preventing heart problems and strokes. It is a special dietary fiber that has a remarkable water-binding and gel-forming capacity to clean out the digestive tract.

Glucomannan can improve metabolism and food assimilation naturally. It also helps absorb toxic substances produced during digestion. It binds toxic substances and eliminates them before they are absorbed into the blood stream. It will help in obesity, high blood pressure, diabetes, heart disease and stroke.

Golden Seal/Echinacea Extract

Golden Seal contains natural antibiotic properties that will stop infections and kill poisons in the body. It has been used as a substitute for quinine with no after-effects. It is valuable for all catarrhal conditions of the bronchial tubes. It has the ability to heal mucous membranes anywhere in the body. It is one of the best herbs to activate the body's own defense system, to fight off infections.

Echinacea has a natural antibiotic effect and is a powerful gland cleanser, eliminating toxins from the lymphatic system. It is useful for chronic and acute bacterial and viral infections. It stimulates the immune response and helps build resistance to disease. Echinacea is a powerful blood cleanser and aids in the removal of toxins from the blood.

Instant Vitamins

This combination of instant vitamins includes vitamins A, D, C, niacinamide, B1, B2, B6, B12, folic acid, biotin, pantothenic acid and calcium, with rose hips and fructose.

Instant vitamins are absorbed into the system quickly for nutritional benefit. It is especially beneficial to the young and elderly who find it hard to swallow capsules.

Licorice Lozenges with Zinc

These are essential to have on hand for sudden sore throats. They contain licorice root, zinc, oil of anise, peppermint oil and eucalyptus. Zinc has been found very effective in healing a sore throat when used at the very first sign. Licorice root is well known as a healing herb for throat problems as well as laryngitis.

Nutritional Fiber Supplement

This supplement contains natural ingredients to provide fiber and bulk to the diet for a healthy colon. It contains fructose, maltodextrin, soy bran, corn, base, lecithin, cellulose, apple pectin, carrot powder, prune powder, citric acid with natural orange and vanilla flavors.

A nutritional way to keep the gastrointestinal system clean and free from toxins. It will pull heavy metals and additives out of the body before they are absorbed into the blood stream.

Peppermint Oil

Peppermint is the most universally used plant and is considered to be the greatest of all therapeutic remedies. Peppermint oil with hot water (about 10 drops to 2 quarts of water) breathed through the nostrils will open up sinuses. Also can be used as a facial steam bath for acne.

It is used for chills, cholera, colic, coughs, dizziness, earaches, gas, hiccoughs, indigestion, measles, muscle spasms, nausea and vomiting. Externally it can be used for headaches, pain, skin itching, rheumatism and toothaches.

Lecithin

Lecithin helps to regulate metabolism and break down fat and cholesterol and prevent it from adhering to the artery walls. It slows down the aging process and aids in rebuilding brain cells. Lecithin is essential to every cell and organ in the body. It helps fight infections and increases resistance to disease. Lecithin and glucomannan taken together can be of help in preventing heart disease and stroke.

Redmond Clay

Redmond clay is a creamy white clay that has its therapeutic powers from its radioactive abilities. This unique clay has a negative electrical attraction for particles that are positively charged, and most of the toxic poisons in the body are positively charged.

It is used externally as a drawing poultice and has antibiotic and antiseptic properties. It can be used for acne and all skin problems, bee stings, bug bites, burns, pain, swellings, tumors and varicose veins.

Rice Bran Syrup

Natural nutritional, yeast-free B-complex vitamins. They are essential for overall health. The B-complex vitamins are lacking in the average American diet. They are essential for brain and nervous system disorders. Rice bran syrup contains choline and inositol--two necessary nutrients to strengthen the brain and nerves.

It is used for alcoholism, allergies, anemia, arteriosclerosis, arthritis, constipation, diabetes, depression, epilepsy, fatigue, heart disease, hypoglycemia, hysteria, infertility, insomnia, irritability, lung diseases, mental illness, multiple sclerosis, obesity, parasites, senility, stress, wound healing.

Spirulina

Spirulina contains extra lysine, methionine and tryptophan. It contains protein, vitamins, minerals, chlorophyll and RNA and DNA. This food supplement is rich in vitamin A and B-complex and very rich in chlorophyll. It contains the highest amount of B-12 of any other plant food and twice as much as beef liver. It is very rich in protein which is easily digested and assimilated. It helps in illness to supply protein to rebuild cells. It contains potassium for adrenal energy and muscle strength. It helps to remove toxic metals and additives from the system.

It contains thyroxine and amino acids normally produced by the thyroid gland to stimulate metabolism. It is beneficial to the immune system. It contains phenylalanine and tyrosine (two amino acids that feed the brain and affect mood swing). It promotes a feeling of well-being. It has the ability to balance the body's electrical impulses.

Stevia

Another wonderful herb from South America, along with Pau D'Arco. This nutritious herb is three hundred times sweeter than white sugar, and a lot more nourishing. Stevia can be beneficial when craving sweets. It is especially useful for those with candida or PMS, where such an uncontrollable urge for sweets exists. Stevia is an excellent way to satisfy these cravings.

Stevia creates no side effects from its consumption--which cannot be said for other sugar substitutes currently on the market. Be patient, take your time and you will become acquainted with its taste and have a healthier body because of it.

Tea Tree Oil

Tea tree oil has been known for years for its beneficial healing properties. It has been used by the dental and medical professions as an effective germicide. It is also a disinfectant and fungicide. It prevents infections, aids in healing and acts as a local anesthetic to relieve pain. It has been used in shampoos and scalp lotions. It contains forty-eight natural organic substances that work together to produce its healing powers.

It is used for abrasions, acne, arthritis, asthma, athletes feet, backaches, boils, bronchitis, burns (minor), candida, canker sores, chicken pox, colds, cold sores, cuts emphysema, fingernail (infections), foot baths, fungal infections, gargle, gums (infected), hay fever, headaches (sinus), head congestion, head lice, herpes, insect bites, jock itch, laryngitis, leaches, mouth ulcers (mouth wash), muscle aches, pimples, poison oak and ivy, pyorrhea (mouth wash), psoriasis, rashes, ringworm, scalds, scratches, stinging nettle, sunburn, ticks, thrush and wounds.

Vitamin C (Timed Released)

This essential vitamin (which needs to be supplied in the diet daily), contains a balanced source of vitamin C, which is coated to ensure gradual release over an eight hour period. Time-released vitamins are formulated to release nutrients over a longer period of time. Some doctors feel that vitamin C is better taken in a timed-release formula, for it absorbs slowly and is utilized as it is needed.

13

MEN'S HEALTH

Many men tend to ignore their health until they suffer a heart attack, stroke, cancer or other illnesses which force them to slow down, and think about their life style.

Traditionally, men have been less concerned in the wellness of their bodies than women. Some take better care of their car then they do of their bodies. They make sure the oil is changed regularly, the brakes are checked and only gas goes into the gas tanks. They wouldn't think of putting sand or sugar in their gas tanks. Yet, they think very little of the junk food that they put in their bodies. Men are less likely to watch what they eat, and do not think as much about the nutritional value of food.

Norman Cousins is one man that suffered from a serious collagen illness and took an interest in changing his diet. He found the healing benefits of laughter and the mind and body connection. It was a connective tissue disease that he suffered from and is recorded in his book, "Anatomy of an Illness."

Dr. Anthony J. Sattilaro, M.D. took control of his health when he was told he had prostatic cancer, which spread to several parts of his body, including his skull, right shoulder, sternum, left sixth rib and spine.

He was given between eighteen months and three years to live. At this same time his father was dying of cancer. He resigned himself to a slow agonizing death. After his father's death, he encountered a group of people who told him about a diet that would help reverse cancer. He had nothing to lose so he started a diet consisting of 50% whole grains (such as brown rice, whole wheat, millet, oats and barley), 25% locally grown cooked vegetables, 15% beans and seaweeds and the rest made up of soups and various condiments. He also was encouraged to think positively.

About three weeks after he began the dietary regimen, the back pain he had suffered for more than two years completely disappeared, and he stopped taking the pain relievers. After six months on this regime blood tests showed no sign of cancer. He describes his ordeal in his book, "Living Well Naturally."

Men are becoming more aware of health than ever before, because of the research and knowledge available. Men often suffer from diseases caused by poor diet, improper assimilation of essential nutrients and of poor elimination of toxic waste material. Worry, stress and lack of proper rest contribute to men's poor health.

Many men would like a magic pill that would restore their mental and physical capacities. However they do not consider that their eating and living habits have a profound effect on their sexuality. It has long been established in the natural health field that good health and active sex life go hand in hand.

Exercise and good nutrition can help prevent some common ailments. It can help prevent depression, the desire to overeat, and weight gain.

It helps keep the joints and muscles flexible to help prevent arthritis and other joint diseases. It reduces build-up fatty deposits and toxins. It increases circulation to improve the circulatory system health, and lower blood pressure. Exercise helps increase resistance to disease and strengthens muscle tone.

GLANDULAR HEALTH

ADRENAL---Healthy adrenals are necessary for normal sex drive. Malfunction of the adrenal glands can lead to atrophy of prostate testis and other glands. Adrenal exhaustion causes fatigue, muscle weakness, low blood sugar, poor concentration and poor sex drive. Licorice root is revitalizing to the adrenals. Vitamins A, C, B complex, especially pantothenic acid (vitamin B5) Capsicum, Ginseng, Ginkgo, Hawthorn, Suma.

GONADS---The male sex glands need proper nutrition. Minerals such as manganese, selenium and zinc. High amounts of zinc are needed in the testes. Manganese is necessary for sex drive and semen efficiency. Vitamin E is essential for the sex glands. B complex vitamin are deficient in the typical American diet, especially folic acid and B6.

PITUITARY---Secretes gonadotrophic hormones. These hormones control sperm production and male sex hormones. A high concentration of zinc are found in the pituitary. High amounts of vitamin E are concentrated in the pituitary. When vitamin E and zinc are deficient in the diet, it affects the sex glands as well as the pituitary.

THYROID---This gland is involved in the sex drive. If the thyroid is low it causes lethargy, fatigue, the tendency to gain weight, and low sex drive. The thyroid needs iodine which is found in kelp and dulse.

PROSTATE PROBLEMS

The prostate is located between the urinary tract, the bladder and the rectum. The colon, when not kept clean, collects waste material and presses against the prostate and bladder and can cause irritation and infections. The waste material can also enter the blood stream and cause weakness in the prostate.

A cleansing program is essential to keep the prostate healthy. Eliminate coffee, alcoholic tobacco, caffeine drinks and drink lots of pure water.

Anger, hate, stress and deep resentments can contribute to prostate problems.

Prostate enlargement is common in about 1/3 of men between the ages of 40 and 60. It is known as benign prostatic hyperplasia (B.P.H.). The prostate becomes enlarged and presses against the urethral canal. This back up in the kidneys will obstruct the bladder outlet and causes retention of urine.

Prostatitis is an inflammation of the prostate gland. It can block the urine flow. It can cause pain and frequent urination with a burning sensation and blood or pus in the urine.

Prostate cancer is common among men over sixty. It is not easily detected in the early stages. There is a marked decrease of zinc in those with cancer of the prostate.

A high fiber diet using whole grains, seeds (especially pumpkin), nuts, sprouts, fruit, vegetables and nutritional supplements is essential for a healthy prostate.

Echinacea is an excellent herb for enlargement and weakness of the prostate gland. Cayenne for circulation; kelp is rich in minerals and helps clean the prostate; Saw Palmetto helps to reduce inflammation, pain and swelling. Parsley, and herbal combinations are good to ease urination; they are a natural diuretic. Burdock is excellent for enlarged prostate. Vitamins A and E, C, selenium and zinc help prevent cancer-causing free radicals in the cells.

VITAMINS FOR MEN'S HEALTH

Vitamin A and D promote liver health, heals mucus membranes, assists in the body's natural production of steroids. Protects against free radicals destroying the cells.

Vitamin B complex is essential for healthy nerves, energy and is beneficial for anxiety and depression. B12 prevents nerve damage, maintains fertility and is necessary for normal growth, also helps in digestion. B2 helps sustain youthfulness and increases life span, protects against disease, promotes appetite, digestion, assimilation and elimination. B6 increases energy in brain and nerves, protects against stress and controls cholesterol metabolism. All B vitamins are necessary to nourish, protect, and heal all organs of the body.

Vitamin C and bioflavonoids--Increases sperm count and mobility. Helps calcium and other minerals to absorb. Heals infections, promotes healthy blood vessels, and capillaries, protects against viruses and germs.

Vitamin E--Iodine and E work together for absorption. An antioxidant to protect against free radical damage. Vitamin E nourishes and protects the glands. Promotes normal adrenal function and glandular activity. Increases hormone production and is necessary for reproduction. Promotes the function of the sexual glands.

Vitamin F or Essential Fatty Acids--works with vitamin E to reduce the amount of urine that is retained in the bladder after urinating. EFA's are the building blocks from which prostaglandins are made. Prostaglandin are hormone-like substances that regulate every organ, tissue and cell in the human body at a basic cellular level. They insulate the nerves. Strengthens hormone production. Helps to dissolve brown body fat (the fat that lies deep in the body and surrounds the organs such at the heart, kidneys and adrenals. Found in borage, evening primrose oil, black current oil, Salmon oil.

MINERALS FOR MEN'S HEALTH

Calcium--Necessary for healthy nerves, bones and muscles. Calms nerves, strengthens heart muscles, promotes healing, and increases resistance to infections. Calcium works with magnesium, sulfur and zinc along with B12, C and inositol for healthy sperm, and sexual organs. Horsetail and oatstraw are high in silicon which is necessary in calcium assimilation.

Chlorine--Expels waste, purifies and disinfects against germs and viruses. Helps regulate acid and alkaline balance of blood and hormone distribution.

Iodine--Essential for regulating the thyroid gland, manufacturing the hormone thyroxine to control the metabolism of the body. It affects growth rate and helps burn excess fat.

Magnesium--Works with calcium in the production of sex hormones. Helps in stressful situations.

POTASSIUM--Prevents cancer and tumors from growing. A healing mineral that protects the body and keeps it healthy. It repairs the liver and aids in waste elimination.

SELENIUM--It is important for the testes and is believed necessary for sperm production. It works with vitamin E as an antioxidant to protect against toxins. Helps to prevent chromosome breakage, which causes birth defects.

SULPHUR--Essential in the stimulation of egg and sperm production. Necessary for having children. It promotes growth, essential for protein absorption. Must be balanced with phosphorus for proper assimilation.

ZINC--Essential for health of the prostate gland. It helps to manufacture male hormones and proper development of the genital organs. Silicon and zinc are a valuable beauty aid promoting growth of hair.

HERBS FOR MEN'S HEALTH

Herbal plants radiate energy that can promote cellular growth. Herbs help the body heal itself. Herbs do not heal; the body heals itself when given the proper nourishment. Herbs build, nourish and help to maintain good health.

Herbal formulas for men should contain the following: Damiana, Fo-ti, Ginseng, Gotu Kola, Ho-Shou-Wu, Licorice root, Sarsaparilla, Saw Palmetto.

BEE POLLEN--Contains concentrations of vital nutrients, rich in vitamins, minerals, and amino acids. Good for healthy sex glands. Rich in magnesium, zinc and vitamin F (essential fatty acids), stimulates sex hormones.

BURDOCK, CHAPARRAL, BUCKTHORN, GOLDEN SEAL, ECHINACEA-- help to keep the blood clean and pure. Prevent deposits in the joints, bones and veins. Keep the lymphatic system clean and prevent diseases.

CAYENNE, HAWTHORN AND PRICKLY ASH BARK--Nourishes and protects the heart and veins. Promotes healing, provides nutrition for the heart.

DAMIANA--Increases sperm count and balances hormones. Acts as an aphrodisiac, protects the male sex glands, tonic for the nervous system. Good for weakness and exhaustion. Restores natural sexual function.

DANDELION--Improves liver function and bile production. Purifies the blood and liver. Rich in vitamins, minerals, protein, choline, insulin and pectin.

EPHEDRA--The action of ephedra is a different stimulant than caffeine. In experimental and clinical studies it promotes metabolism and decreases appetite. A slow metabolism is caused by the lack of stimulation by the sympathetic nervous system.

Ephedra promotes weight loss because of its thermogenic and fat metabolizing effects.

GINSENG--Research has proven that ginseng has an adaptogenic and tonic effect. It emits a mitogenetic force field which stimulates glandular activity by increasing hormonal production.

Good for blood pressure, relieves impotence, and lowers cholesterol.

HOPS, SCULLCAP, PASSION FLOWER, VALERIAN ROOT--All of the nervine herbs help strengthen and nourish the nervous system. Good for insomnia and relaxing the body. They relieve depression and promote a feeling of well-being.

Hormonal Herbs--Contains substances necessary for men and women to enable the body to produce its own hormones. Some of the popular ones are Black Cohosh, Sarsaparilla, Ginseng, Licorice, False Unicorn, Blessed Thistle, and Squaw Vine.

Licorice Root - Contains constituents that stimulate natural steroids. Revitalizes the adrenal glands. It has demulcent and anti-inflammatory properties which help in cold, catarrh and bronchitis. Good for ulcers and gastritis.

Sarsaparilla—Balances glands, increases metabolic rate, and stimulates hormone function in men and women. It contains properties to promote the hormone testosterone.

Saw Palmetto—Feeds the glands. It reduces an enlarged prostate, normalizes urinary frequency. Improves male sexual function.

Wood Betony, Feverfew, Cayenne, Gotu Kola— Helps in headaches, and tension. They are found in herbal formulas with other nourishing herbs.

Yucca—Stimulates the body to produce its own cortisone by supplying materials needed to be manufactured in the adrenal gland. It helps all glands of the body.

14

WOMEN'S HEALTH

Most women are more aware and sensitive to their health problems than men. They seem to be more spiritually, emotionally and mentally in tune with their bodies because they have a monthly menstrual cycle to contend with from an early age. The reproductive organs play an important role in the entire life of every woman. Their functions should not cause pain and discomfort. Menstruation is a from of body cleansing of material, preparing for a potential pregnancy. In addition, each month many toxins are eliminated with the flow, which acts to purify the blood. This is why it is important that a woman should learn ways to experience a normal, natural monthly cycle.

HORMONAL IMBALANCE

High levels of the hormone estrogen have been linked to PMS and other health problems. Excess estrogen acts as a stimulant to the central nervous system and contributes to many women's ailments. Women's livers are known to be more sluggish than men's in removing toxins from the body.

Estrogen accumulates in the body; estrogen pills and tranquilizers add to the liver's burden. Poor nutrition causes the liver to function improperly.

Normally, the liver treats estrogen like a poison, removing it immediately from the body. Poor nutrition, drugs, and other bad living habits allows bad estrogen to build up to reach high levels and cause physical and mental problems.

Tests have shown that the flow of estrogen through the liver can be turned off or on by providing B complex vitamins in the diet. When excess estrogen is built up in the liver, the liver is unable to detoxify itself and stress is created in the body, (from water retention to severe mental anguish). Excess estrogen has a strong effect on women in various ways. Changes in hormone levels are noticeable anywhere from four days to two weeks before the period begins. Definite drops in the pituitary and ovarian hormones have been measured, which may be the reason for the emotional reaction during this time.

MALNUTRITION AND CONSTIPATION

The blood is the life of the body, and every cell is nourished or poisoned through the blood. It needs to be kept clean and pure so it can carry nutrients through the system and carry off all waste material. Constipation puts pressure on the uterus and causes pain. It also is the cause of toxic blood. A change of diet and keeping the bowels clean and open can prevent women's problems. A lower bowel formula is necessary to feed, strengthen and stimulate proper bowel function.

STRESS AND FIBROSITIS

Stress affects our entire body and weakens the immune system. Stress depletes nutrients from our system. W need to replace nutrients to strengthen our immune system so we can properly handle stress. Vitamins A and C with bioflavonoids should be used daily. The nervine herbs will build and feed the nervous system. The body craves and demands food to nourish it and if it isn't satisfied puts more stress upon the body. This can cause irritability and emotional problems as well as disease.

One syndrome that causes chronic muscle aches, pains and stiffness and a tightening up of our inner body is fibrositis. It is also called chronic muscle syndrome. It has many symptoms and has been around for many years. It has been called muscular rheumatism, fibromyositis, and tension myalgia. Some of the common complaints are: fatigue and exhaustion, tension or migraine-type headaches, insomnia, joint swelling, tension and poor stress tolerance and anxiety and depression. With this condition we need to improve our nutrition, learn to control the stress in our lives, exercise and massage therapy, and learn to rest and relax.

CALCIUM AND FEMALE PROBLEMS

Blood calcium drops ten days prior to menstruation. It happens when the ovaries are not producing much estrogen or progesterone and continues until even after menstruation starts. A calcium decrease causes tension, headaches, nervousness, insomnia, and depression. Diet has a lot to do with calcium absorption. It is usually what you are eating that causes calcium loss. Sugar, soft drinks, caffeine, alcohol, meat especially beef and a poor diet can deplete calcium and other essential minerals. An excellent herbal combination should contain horsetail and oatstraw. They contain silicon, which helps the body utilize calcium.

THE OVARIES AND PITUITARY GLANDS

The glands controlling femininity, emotions, and sexuality are the ovaries (one on either side of the uterus) and the pituitary (located in the brain).

The ovaries produce estrogen and progesterone in about a 28-day cycle. Estrogen is responsible for breast development, increasing bone and protein deposition and it stimulates hair growth on pubis and armpits.

Progesterone prepares the uterus for pregnancy and the breasts for lactation. Progesterone is secreted in the last half of the ovarian cycle and during pregnancy and in larger quantities by the placenta. Still, estrogen is more potent than progesterone.

When the body is fed properly the gland works without any problems, but when sugar, high meat diet, and white flour products, are eaten, it depletes nutrients from the body and this can cause an imbalance in the system.

Vitamin E is known as the "fertility vitamin", vital to the sex glands of both male and female. It is felt the health of these glands is related to the condition of the brain in old age.

The B-complex vitamins are very important for women. A sufficient amount allows the liver to control the level of estrogen in the blood. It is considered the bad estrogen. Too much of this bad estrogen in the blood stream causes many mental and physical problems. It creates a lower threshold to stress, nervous tension, water retention and abnormal sugar tolerance. Some women become aggressive, hostile and assertive due to excess estrogen in the body. Birth control pills cause excess estrogen to accumulate. An herbal formula designed to clean the liver should contain Dandelion Root and Red Beet Root along with other vital herbs.

The pituitary gland is called the master gland because it affects the entire glandular system. An underactive pituitary gland can upset major portions of the body's chemistry and will often produce sugar cravings. This becomes a vicious cycle to stronger sugar cravings that can lead to hypoglycemia.

Pituitary hormones also help to maintain water balance. A weak pituitary causes frequent urination, swollen ankles, bags under the eyes and a general bloated appearance. It is estimated that 88% of women have underactive pituitary glands. The growth-monitoring portion of the pituitary gland contains seven to ten times the bromine concentration of any other organ. Kelp and dulce contain traces of bromine, as do mussels, sea water and animal glands.

Lack of potassium and sodium can also ruin pituitary production. Potassium herbs are dulce, irish moss, valerian, stevia, scullcap saffron, red clover, parsley, licorice, horsetail, hops and garlic.

Natural sodium is more easily utilized and

excreted by the body than table salt (sodium chloride). Sodium herbs are: alfalfa, chickweed, buchu, burdock, gotu kola, saffron, sarsaparilla, rosehips, parsley, licorice, and dandelion.

MINERALS ESSENTIAL FOR WOMEN'S HEALTH

CALCIUM- The body's most abundant mineral is calcium. Important minerals for women are calcium, phosphorus, and magnesium. Phosphorus is the second most abundant mineral in the body.

Blood calcium drops ten days prior to menstruation. It happens when the ovaries are not producing much estrogen or progesterone and continues until even after menstruation starts. A calcium decrease causes tension, headaches, nervousness, insomnia, and depression. Magnesium and vitamin D aid in calcium absorption. Calcium and magnesium are also very helpful in eliminating cramps. An herbal formula for calcium assimilation should contain horsetail and oatstraw.

PHOSPHORUS- The second most abundant mineral in the body is phosphorus. It works along with calcium in the bones. It is found in every cell in the body. If there is an imbalance of phosphorus calcium can be lost. Lack of phosphorus in the body effect the brain and emotions. It could cause weakness, fatigue, criticism, and slow oxygenation. It is a mineral essential for women.

MAGNESIUM- An important mineral for women. It increases B-complex absorption and helps the body diminish excess estrogen in the blood stream.

This nutrient relieves cramps, calms the nervous system and is a blood-clotting agent. It prevents spasms in uterus walls, leg muscles and eliminates irritability and depression. It helps prevent constipation and indigestion.

ZINC- This trace mineral is essential for many functions. It is instrumental in stabilizing blood sugar levels and helps the body regulate and release "prostaglandins" (substances which help control cramping). It also aids in the balancing of hormones.

IRON- It is very vital to the body and carries oxygen to the tissues. It can be depleted during menstruation if the woman is not eating properly. Iron helps prevent anemia. It helps when there is fatigue, weakness, and depression stemming from low red blood cell count. Vitamin C helps the body assimilate iron.

CHROMIUM- This helps stabilize blood sugar levels, much like zinc does. It works closely with insulin to accomplish this. Lack of this mineral can affect atherosclerosis.

IODINE- This mineral helps the thyroid stay healthy and aids in the production of "thyroxine." This substance is an aid to balance hormone levels. Its function is to keep estrogen levels from becoming too high. This helps the body regulate menstrual periods and prevent water retention.

MANGANESE- This mineral is vital for normal reproduction and the mammary glands. It is important to prevent osteoporosis. It is concentrated in the tissues of the bones, liver, pituitary gland, kidneys, pancreas and intestines.

POTASSIUM- This "electrolyte" helps regulate water balance in the tissues. Too much sodium chloride will cause a potassium deficiency and promote water retention. Diuretics wash potassium out of the body.

SELENIUM- It is a mineral necessary for a strong immune system. It is excellent to prevent menstrual cramps and breast tenderness.

VITAMINS FOR WOMEN'S HEALTH

VITAMIN A- This vitamin is responsible for stimulating antibody production, thus reducing the risk of infections. It also helps maintain the health of the mucous membranes, our inner skin. This includes the lining of the reproductive organs. Endocrine glands associated with the reproductive cycle need vitamin A to function properly. It helps alleviate monthly skin disorders.

VITAMIN C- It promotes the healing of cells and tissues. Vitamin C helps alleviate stress because it fortifies the adrenal (stress) gland function. The "C-complex" includes bioflavonoids, which strengthen capillary walls and prevent hemorrhaging. Vitamin C is a natural diuretic. It helps regulate menstrual flow and relieves pain associated with it. This vitamin does not store in the body. It is needed as a supplement each day, to prevent stress, air pollution, infections and etc.

VITAMIN E- This is a very essential nutrient for the reproductive system. It has several functions. Among them are easing breast tenderness and alleviating fibrocystic breast disease, equalizing blood circulation, reducing fluid retention, eliminating cramps. Vitamin E is important both to the adequate production and proper metabolism of the sex hormones. It helps prevent heart problems.

VITAMIN D-The primary responsibility of vitamin D is to help the body absorb calcium properly. It also assists in calming the nerves and aids in promoting restful sleep.

B-COMPLEX-The B vitamins play a major and vital role in preventing women's problems. Tests have shown that the amount of estrogen metabolized by the liver can be controlled through sufficient intake of B vitamins. The B's are crucial, therefore, to regulating estrogen and preventing the anguish caused by an excessive amount of this hormone in the body as well as affecting the brain. B-complex vitamins help change estrogen to a less harmful and potent hormone called "estriol." If the diet is deficient in B vitamins, estrogen may accumulate in the breast and uterine tissue, precipitating the risk of cancer. B's are essential to prevent fatigue, sugar cravings, weight fluctuation and bloating. Lack of B-2 can also cause depression and fatigue, as well as loss of appetite for natural food and irritability. The B vitamins especially linked to estrogen conversion are choline, inositol, lecithin, B-6 and B-12. The first three are particularly useful in preventing fatty deposits in the liver. Lack of B-6 can cause female problems. Folic acid is a very essential B vitamin which strengthens the reproductive system.

HERBS FOR WOMEN'S HEALTH

BLACK COHOSH- Useful in estrogen production and ovulation. It helps enable transport of estrogen throughout the body. It strengthens the uterus. It is good for irregular or scanty menstruation with muscular aches and pains. It helps during menopause.

BLESSED THISTLE-It increases production of mother's milk. It balances hormones and can help with infertility. It is a tonic and blood purifier. Good for menopause, to balance hormones.

BLUE COHOSH-It is used in the last week of pregnancy to stimulate contractions. It has been used for hysteria and uterine inflammation. It will also increase the flow of milk. It is used in herbal female formulas.

BURDOCK-It increases sweat, urination and bile to clean the body. It acts as a blood purifier. It restores liver function. It promotes kidney function to eliminate harmful acids. Its insulin content aids the pituitary gland in releasing an ample supply of protein to help balance hormones.

CRAMP BARK-It is good for congestion and hardening of the liver. A valuable herb to help prevent nervous disorders in pregnancy. Helps in after-pain and cramps. It is a uterine sedative and relaxes the muscles. Helpful in the cramping pains of pregnancy which occur in the legs and calves.

DONG QUAI-An excellent woman's tonic. It is useful for muscle cramps and nervousness. It helps to balance hormones. Contains vitamin E. It helps in premenstrual syndrome and menopausal symptoms. It is beneficial for candida and enhances the immune system; promotes healthy arteries and blood vessels.

FALSE UNICORN-It stimulates the reproductive organs in men and women. It is used in herbal combination to correct almost all problems of the reproductive organs. It is effective during menopause because of its effect on uterine disorders, headaches and depression.

FEVERFEW-This is considered a woman's herb. It strengthens the womb, and helps expel the afterbirth. It promotes the menses, and calms the nerves. It helps in inflammation, and migraine headaches.

HORSETAIL-Along with oatstraw and comfrey are calcium herbs. The silica in horsetail converts to calcium in the body. Calcium is necessary for nerve sheath, veins and artery walls, bones, teeth, nails and healthy hair.

LICORICE ROOT-It nourishes and feeds the adrenal cortical tissue. It helps stimulate hormone production. It is said to increase fertility during ovulation. It increases energy production.

RED CLOVER-An excellent tonic for the nervous system. It cleans the blood and liver. It tends to dry mucous membranes and helps vaginal infections.

RED RASPBERRY-An astringent and tonic that benefits the uterine wall in stabilizing excessive flow and also in relieving pain. It strengthens the uterus for safe and easy delivery. It relieves vomiting, provides energy. It equalizes and restores balance of circulation in the body.

SARSAPARILLA-It helps in progesterone stimulation, which sustains pregnancy and relaxes muscles. It is a natural diuretic and digestive aid.

WILD YAM-A valuable herb used in glandular formulas. It helps balance hormones. It contains ingredients to simulate natural steroid hormones. It acts as a antispasmodic for menstrual cramps and muscle aches and pains.

YELLOW DOCK-Rich in organic iron. Lack of iron can cause dizziness, headaches, tiredness, lack of endurance, shortness of breath and depression.

NERVINE HERBS-Chamomile, Hops, Passion Flower, Lady's Slipper, Scullcap, St. Johnswort and Valerian all help in strengthening the nervous system and prevent wearing away of the nerve sheath. They are soothing and calming to help women cope with the stress of daily living.

OTHER BOOKS BY LOUISE TENNEY

Published by
Woodland Health Books

TODAY'S HERBAL HEALTH

TODAY'S HEALTHY EATING

TODAY'S HEALTH SERIES

> #1 *Candida Albicans: A Nutritional Approach*
> #2 *The Immune System: A Nutritional Approach*
> #3 *PMS Syndrome: A Nutritional Approach*
> #4 *Allergies: A Nutritional Approach*
> #5 *Stress: A Nutritional Approach*
> #6 *AIDS: A Nutritional Approach*
> #7 *Herpes: A Nutritional Approach*
> #8 *Weight Control: A Nutritional Approach*

Louise Tenney is also editor of a newsletter, published monthly called TODAY'S HERBS.

BIBLIOGRAPHY

Balch, James F. Jr., M.D., F.A.C.S. and Phyllis A. Balch, N.C., *Nutritional Outline For The Professional (and The Wise Man).*

Chaitow, Leon, N.C., D.O., M.B.N.O.A., *School Of Natural Healing.*

Colbin, Annemarie, *Food And Healing.*

Fuchs, Nan Kathryn, Ph.D., *The Nutrition Detective.*

Hoffmann, David, *The Holisitic Herbal.*

Hoffman, Dr. Jay M., *The Missing Link.*

Griffin, LaDean, *Health In The Space Age.*

Malstrom, N.D., M.T., *Own Your Own Body.*

Millet, Edward Milo, *Herbal Aid.*

Montagna, F. Joseph, P.D.R. *People's Desk Refernce, Traditional Herbal Formulas,* Vol. 1 and 2.

Santillo, Humbart, B.S., M.H., *Natural Healing With Herbs.*

Tenney, Louise, M.H., *Today's Healthy Eating, Today's Herbal Health, Today's Health Series*, Volumes 1 through 8; *Today's Herbs*, Newsletter.

Tierra, Michael, C.A., N.D. *The Way Of Herbs.*

Weiner, Michael A., Ph.D., *Maximum Immunity.*

INDEX

A

B

C

D

E

H

I

M

N